Insuring America's Health

Principles and Recommendations

Committee on the Consequences of Uninsurance

Board on Health Care Services

INSTITUTE OF MEDICINE
OF THE NATIONAL ACADEMIES

THE NATIONAL ACADEMIES PRESS
Washington, D.C.
www.nap.edu

THE NATIONAL ACADEMIES PRESS • 500 Fifth Street, N.W. • **Washington, DC 20001**

NOTICE: The project that is the subject of this report was approved by the Governing Board of the National Research Council, whose members are drawn from the councils of the National Academy of Sciences, the National Academy of Engineering, and the Institute of Medicine. The members of the committee responsible for the report were chosen for their special competences and with regard for appropriate balance.

Support for this project was provided by The Robert Wood Johnson Foundation. The views presented in this report are those of the Institute of Medicine Committee on the Consequences of Uninsurance and are not necessarily those of the funding agency.

International Standard Book Number 0-309-09105-5 (Book)
International Standard Book Number 0-309-52826-7 (PDF)
Library of Congress Control Number 2003114736

Additional copies of this report are available for sale from the National Academies Press, 2101 Constitution Avenue, N.W., Box 285, Washington, DC 20055. Call (800) 624-6242 or (202) 334-3313 (in the Washington metropolitan area); Internet, http://www.nap.edu.

For more information about the Institute of Medicine, visit the IOM home page at **www.iom.edu**.

The serpent has been a symbol of long life, healing, and knowledge among almost all cultures and religions since the beginning of recorded history. The serpent adopted as a logotype by the Institute of Medicine is a relief carving from ancient Greece, now held by the Staatliche Museen in Berlin.

*"Knowing is not enough; we must apply.
Willing is not enough; we must do."*
                                    —Goethe

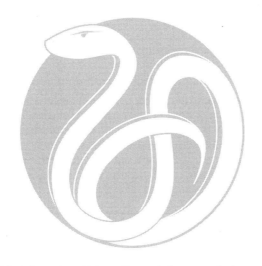

INSTITUTE OF MEDICINE
OF THE NATIONAL ACADEMIES

Shaping the Future for Health

THE NATIONAL ACADEMIES
Advisers to the Nation on Science, Engineering, and Medicine

The **National Academy of Sciences** is a private, nonprofit, self-perpetuating society of distinguished scholars engaged in scientific and engineering research, dedicated to the furtherance of science and technology and to their use for the general welfare. Upon the authority of the charter granted to it by the Congress in 1863, the Academy has a mandate that requires it to advise the federal government on scientific and technical matters. Dr. Bruce M. Alberts is president of the National Academy of Sciences.

The **National Academy of Engineering** was established in 1964, under the charter of the National Academy of Sciences, as a parallel organization of outstanding engineers. It is autonomous in its administration and in the selection of its members, sharing with the National Academy of Sciences the responsibility for advising the federal government. The National Academy of Engineering also sponsors engineering programs aimed at meeting national needs, encourages education and research, and recognizes the superior achievements of engineers. Dr. Wm. A. Wulf is president of the National Academy of Engineering.

The **Institute of Medicine** was established in 1970 by the National Academy of Sciences to secure the services of eminent members of appropriate professions in the examination of policy matters pertaining to the health of the public. The Institute acts under the responsibility given to the National Academy of Sciences by its congressional charter to be an adviser to the federal government and, upon its own initiative, to identify issues of medical care, research, and education. Dr. Harvey V. Fineberg is president of the Institute of Medicine.

The **National Research Council** was organized by the National Academy of Sciences in 1916 to associate the broad community of science and technology with the Academy's purposes of furthering knowledge and advising the federal government. Functioning in accordance with general policies determined by the Academy, the Council has become the principal operating agency of both the National Academy of Sciences and the National Academy of Engineering in providing services to the government, the public, and the scientific and engineering communities. The Council is administered jointly by both Academies and the Institute of Medicine. Dr. Bruce M. Alberts and Dr. Wm. A. Wulf are chair and vice chair, respectively, of the National Research Council.

www.national-academies.org

COMMITTEE ON THE CONSEQUENCES OF UNINSURANCE

★Served from September 2000 to December 2002.

IOM Staff

Wilhelmine Miller, Project Co-director
Dianne Miller Wolman, Project Co-director
Lynne Page Snyder, Program Officer
Tracy McKay,★ Research Associate
Ryan Palugod, Senior Project Assistant

Consultant

Cheryl Ulmer, Writer

★Served until August 2003.

Reviewers

This report has been reviewed in draft form by individuals chosen for their diverse perspectives and technical expertise, in accordance with procedures approved by the National Research Council's Report Review Committee. The purpose of this independent review is to provide candid and critical comments that will assist the institution in making its published report as sound as possible and to ensure that the report meets institutional standards for objectivity, evidence, and responsiveness to the study charge. The review comments and draft manuscript remain confidential to protect the integrity of the deliberative process. We wish to thank the following individuals for their review of this report:

Sheila Burke, Smithsonian's Under Secretary for American Museums and National Programs, Smithsonian Institution, Washington, DC.

Robert Cunningham, Deputy Editor, Health Affairs, Bethesda, MD.

Helen Darling, President, Washington Business Group on Health, Washington, DC.

Michael M. E. Johns, Executive Vice President for Health Affairs, Emory University, Atlanta, GA.

Charles N. Kahn, III, President, American Federation of Hospitals, Washington, DC.

Catherine McLaughlin, Director, Economic Research Initiatives on the Uninsured, University of Michigan, Ann Arbor.

Mark Pauly, Bendheim Professor, The Wharton School, University of Pennsylvania, Philadelphia.

Trish Riley, Executive Director, National Academy for State Health Policy, Portland, ME.

Diane Rowland, Executive Vice President, Kaiser Family Foundation, Washington, DC.

Leonard Schaeffer, Chief Executive Officer, WellPoint Health Networks, Inc., Thousand Oaks, CA.

Rosemary Stevens, Stanley I. Sheerr Professor in Arts and Sciences, Emerita, University of Pennsylvania, Philadelphia.

Although the reviewers listed above have provided many constructive comments and suggestions, they were not asked to endorse the conclusions or recommendations nor did they see the final draft of the report before its release. The review of this report was overseen by **Hugh H. Tilson, Clinical Professor, School of Public Health, University of North Carolina, Chapel Hill,** and **Joseph P. Newhouse, John D. MacArthur Professor of Health Policy and Management, Harvard University**. Appointed by the National Research Council and Institute of Medicine, they were responsible for making certain that an independent examination of this report was carried out in accordance with institutional procedures and that all review comments were carefully considered. Responsibility for the final content of this report rests entirely with the authoring committee and the institution.

Foreword

Insuring America's Health: Principles and Recommendations concludes the series of groundbreaking reports by the Institute of Medicine and its Committee on the Consequences of Uninsurance. The previous five Committee reports, issued between October 2001 and June 2003, have established both a broader conceptual framework and a new empirical evidence base with which to assess the implications of our nation's policies regarding health insurance and of the lack of coverage for one out of every seven Americans.

Beginning with *Coverage Matters*, which dispelled common misconceptions about who lacks health insurance, why, and the access implications of being uninsured, the Committee's reports examine multiple facets of the problem of uninsurance and systematically address questions relevant for public policy. *Care Without Coverage: Too Little, Too Late* documents the serious health risks that the lack of coverage poses for adults. *Health Insurance Is a Family Matter* extends this examination of health outcomes to those of pregnant women and infants and children, and considers the psychosocial and financial impacts that the lack of health insurance for any family member has on the whole family. The Committee's fourth report, *A Shared Destiny: Community Effects of Uninsurance*, extends the scope of analysis even further, to conceptualize and determine how the presence of uninsured residents might affect the health, health care, and social and economic life of neighborhoods, towns, cities, and rural areas. Notably, this report includes an original study of community-level effects of uninsurance on the availability of hospital services and hospital financial margins. In *Hidden Costs, Value Lost*, its fifth report, the Committee presents an innovative assessment of the economic implications of the lack of health insurance across society. This analysis considers the economic value lost to the nation in terms of the poorer health and shorter lives of uninsured Americans relative to the cost of providing health care services to those without coverage comparable to what insured people enjoy.

Anyone who has become familiar with the wealth of timely information and the thoughtfully presented analytic discussions in these reports on the consequences of uninsurance is in a much better position to join in the national policy debate concerning the extension of health insurance coverage. Once again, after a decade during which the issue was effectively tabled, the debate revolves less around whether or not universal health insurance coverage is a good idea than it does about the best way to accomplish that goal. *Insuring America's Health: Principles and Recommendations*, the Committee's final installment in its series, collects the Committee's insights developed over the course of this project and demonstrates how this understanding of the virtues and advantages of health insurance can be used to evaluate and make choices among reform strategies.

I commend this volume to you as a most useful tool with which to approach the task of reforming American health insurance.

Harvey V. Fineberg, M.D., Ph.D.
President, Institute of Medicine
January 2004

Preface

Insuring America's Health: Principles and Recommendations is the sixth and last report in a series by the Institute of Medicine Committee on the Consequences of Uninsurance. The Committee began this project three years ago with the intent to consolidate the ever-growing evidence on uninsurance effects and to communicate our findings to policy makers, the media, and the public. Our hope was that these reports would stimulate a more informed public debate and a reexamination of the issue of financial access to health care. At the time the Committee began its work in 2000, about 40 million Americans lacked any health insurance coverage, despite the strong economy of the previous decade. Since then, another three million individuals have been added to the rolls of the uninsured.

The Committee's first five reports carefully assess and document the nature and severity of the problems resulting from uninsurance. The clinical literature overwhelmingly shows that uninsured people, children as well as adults, suffer worse health and die sooner than those with insurance. Families with even one member who is uninsured lose peace of mind and can become burdened with enormous medical bills. Uninsurance at the community level is associated with financial instability for health care providers and institutions, reduced hospital services and capacity, and significant cuts in public health programs, which may diminish access to certain types of care for all residents, even those who have coverage. The economic vitality of the nation is limited by productivity lost as a result of the poorer health and premature death or disability of uninsured workers. The Committee has estimated that the economic value lost because of poorer health and earlier deaths among uninsured Americans is between $65 billion and $130 billion annually.

Although some of these conclusions from the Committee's research may seem self-evident to those who regularly study this issue, they counter widely held misperceptions about the personal consequences of uninsurance for tens of millions of Americans. The Committee's findings about family impacts, community-level consequences, and the societal costs of uninsurance break new ground on topics that previously received little attention. Each of the reports organizes a wealth of information within a unified conceptual framework to clarify the magnitude, extent, and impacts of this complex and multifaceted problem. The Committee finds the consistency of the evidence, and the scope and scale of its consequences, compelling. Can we afford *not* to cover the uninsured?

Why hasn't more been done to eliminate uninsurance? Could extension of coverage be achieved through incremental expansions of existing programs or through comprehensive reforms? What *should* be done? These questions are examined in detail in this, the final report of the series. A historical review shows that numerous attempts have been made to extend coverage in this country, beginning a century ago, but most of these efforts have been thwarted or fallen short of expectations. On the strength of this experience, the Committee concludes that further efforts to gradually expand coverage through incremental reforms are unlikely to succeed. Instead, the Committee proposes a clear and compelling goal—within 6 years, everyone in the United States should have health insurance. Based on the Committee's evidence and findings in its first five reports, it has crafted a checklist of principles that can be used to assess the adequacy and impact of various models or proposals to cover the uninsured. There are many current proposals for achieving universal coverage; the Committee does not recommend or propound any particular model. However, the Committee's final report, and the findings of its five previous reports, provides an evidence-based framework to consider the pros and cons of current and future proposals to achieve universal coverage. The Committee urges our national leadership to move forward expeditiously.

What happens next is up to policy makers, elected officials, and the American public. In light of the many consequences of uninsurance, and the continuing stress it imposes on the very fabric of America's health care system, this problem can no longer be ignored. Uninsurance can be eliminated, but it will require the support of the public, considerable technical expertise by policy makers, a spirit of compromise among stakeholders, and courage from our elected officials. We firmly believe that universal coverage of the U.S. population is both feasible and imperative.

As co-chairs, we thank our fellow Committee members for sharing so generously of their expertise and time. Their commitment over the duration of this long project has been outstanding. Although the term of the Committee will soon end, our dedication to implementing the recommendations of this report will endure. We look forward to a time in the not-too-distant future when studies of uninsurance no longer will be needed because everyone will be covered.

> Mary Sue Coleman, Ph.D.
> *Co-chair*
> Arthur L. Kellermann, M.D., M.P.H.
> *Co-chair*
> January 2004

Acknowledgments

It is a pleasure to thank the many people who have participated in the development of *Insuring America's Health*, as well as those who have contributed to the work of the Committee over its three-year term.

The members of the Subcommittee on Strategies and Models for Providing Health Insurance prepared this report for the Committee's consensus review and issuance. Shoshanna Sofaer chaired the Subcommittee. Members included Patricia Butler, George Eads, Jack Ebeler, Barbara Matula, Len Nichols, Christopher Queram, Reed Tuckson, Edward Wagner, and Alan Weil. Through intense discussions, in person and by e-mail, they guided staff, particularly in the historical analysis and the design and analyses of the coverage models. Their expertise has been invaluable to the Committee. Writer Cheryl Ulmer served as a consultant to the Committee on this report and throughout the project. Herman Beals and Joanna Rios provided Spanish translation services for the brief summaries of each report.

Presentations by a number of experts provided a wealth of insights and evidence for consideration by the Committee and Subcommittee, and the Committee thanks them for their contributions of time and expertise. Karen Davis, President of the Commonwealth Fund, reviewed federal efforts and options to expand coverage at a meeting of the full Committee in October 2002. Deborah Chollet, Mathematica Policy Research, Rick Curtis, Institute for Health Policy Solutions, Judy Feder, Georgetown University, Vickie Gates, State Coverage Initiatives, AcademyHealth, and Jack Meyer, Economic and Social Research Institute, discussed issues related to coverage expansions at the local, state, regional, and national levels at the Subcommittee's November 2002 meeting in Washington, DC. Irene Ibarra, Alameda Alliance, and Richard Kronick, University of California at San Diego, shared their experiences and research on local expansions at the February 2002 Committee meeting in San Francisco. In addition, the Committee would like to thank Senator Rosalyn Baker of Hawaii, Toni Beddingfield, Dennis Chu, Jeffrey Lazenby, Nina Maruyama, and Karl Polzer for their insights about the experiences of states and localities with coverage expansions.

The depth and comprehensiveness of this project was possible because of a rich research base and a widely published body of literature. Research and analysis of issues related to uninsurance has been facilitated by the support of three key foundations: the Commonwealth Fund, the Kaiser Family Foundation, and The Robert Wood Johnson Foundation. We are grateful for their longstanding and ongoing support of intellectual inquiry on the topic of the uninsured.

The Committee would like to thank the Institute of Medicine (IOM) project staff for their skilled work on *Insuring America's Health*. Project co-director Dianne Wolman served as principal staff to the Subcommittee and coordinated the drafting of the report. Project co-director Wilhelmine Miller advised on and edited multiple drafts. Program officer Lynne Snyder assisted in drafting and editing, particularly Chapter 3. Research associate Tracy McKay conducted literature searches. Senior project assistant Ryan Palugod maintained the project's research database, prepared the manuscript for publication, and managed the logistics of the Committee's travel and meetings. The wholehearted commitment of the entire project team has made possible this three-year project, as well as the high quality of the Committee's products. The IOM Board on Health Care Services, directed by Janet Corrigan, sponsors and provides overall guidance to the Committee.

Over the course of the Committee's work, staff at the IOM and the National Academies have ably and generously supported the production, public release, and dissemination of the Committee's six reports. IOM President Harvey Fineberg, Past President Kenneth Shine, and Executive Officer Susanne Stoiber encouraged and advised the Committee. The Committee also thanks Clyde Behney, Jennifer Bitticks, Jennifer Otten, and Bronwyn Schrecker at the Office of Reports and Communication; Craig Hicks, Bill Kearney, Lauren Morello, Barbara Rice, Bill Skane, and Christine Stencel at the Office of News and Public Affairs; Jim Jensen and Sandra McDermin at the Office of Government and Congressional Affairs; Dorothy Lewis, Rachel Marcus, Will Mason, Ann Merchant, Estelle Miller, Lynn Murphy, Dan Parham, and Sally Stanfield at the National Academies Press; Jennifer Cangco, Teresa Redd, and Gary Walker at the Office of Finance and Administration; Linda Kilroy at the Office of Contracts and Grants; Bill McLeod of the George Brown Library; and Tony Burton and Ann Greiner of the Board on Health Care Services.

The Committee would like to thank The Robert Wood Johnson Foundation for its generous and continued support of the project on the consequences of uninsurance and especially acknowledges The Foundation's president, Risa Lavizzo-Mourey, this project's program officer Anne Weiss, and Linda Bilheimer, David Colby, and Stuart Schear for their interest and assistance with this project.

Finally, the Committee thanks co-chairs Mary Sue Coleman and Arthur Kellermann for their leadership and commitment over the three-year course of the Committee's term.

Contents

Insuring America's Health

Principles and Recommendations

Executive Summary

ABSTRACT

The lack of health insurance for tens of millions of Americans has serious negative consequences and economic costs not only for the uninsured themselves but also for their families, the communities they live in, and the whole country. The situation is dire and expected to worsen. The Committee urges Congress and the Administration to act immediately to eliminate this longstanding problem.

This report offers a framework for the public and policy makers to use as they weigh the pros and cons of various proposals. The framework consists of a set of principles informed by the research and analysis of the five previous reports in this series. The principles are applied to selected coverage prototypes to demonstrate the extent to which various proposals for extending coverage or designing new strategies to eliminate uninsurance would improve the current situation.

The lack of health insurance coverage for a substantial number of Americans has been a public policy problem throughout the past century and particularly over the past three decades. Three years ago, following a decade of strong economic growth but little progress reducing the number of uninsured, the problem was urgent; 39 million people under age 65 reported having been without insurance during the entire previous year.[1] In 2000, the Institute of Medicine (IOM)

---

[1]The estimate of the uninsured is based on the Census Bureau's annual March Current Population Survey (CPS), as are all annual estimates of the uninsured population of the United States presented in this report, unless otherwise noted. The CPS may overestimate the number of uninsured for the entire calendar year and does not account for all who are uninsured for shorter time periods (CBO, 2003). See Chapter 2 for a discussion of who is uninsured, why, and for how long.

formed an expert Committee on the Consequences of Uninsurance to study the issue comprehensively, examining the effects of the lack of health coverage on individuals, families, communities, and the broader society.[2] Now, after a significant economic downturn, 17.2 percent of the population under age 65 is uninsured and the number has grown to over 43 million. One in three Americans were uninsured for a month or more during a two-year period (1996-1997) (Short, 2001). Fewer people have access to coverage at work, more people find the costs of private coverage too expensive, and others lose public coverage because of changed personal circumstances, administrative barriers, and program cutbacks. The situation is even more dire now than when the study began and it is expected to worsen in the foreseeable future because of federal and state budget constraints limiting public coverage programs, increasing costs of health care and insurance premiums, and continuing high rates of unemployment.

WHY SHOULD POLICY MAKERS AND THE PUBLIC CARE ABOUT COVERAGE?

The Committee has conducted an exhaustive review of the scientific evidence on the consequences of uninsurance and finds that having no insurance decreases access to health services and reduced access to health care among the uninsured is associated with poorer health. The lack of coverage is not only associated with negative effects on the uninsured individual but also has implications for the entire family of the uninsured person and the community in which he or she lives, and economic costs to society nationally (IOM, 2001a, 2002a, b, 2003a, b). In short, in a series of five reports **the Committee concluded that:**

• **The number of uninsured individuals under age 65 is large, growing, and has persisted even during periods of strong economic growth.**
• **Uninsured children and adults do not receive the care they need; they suffer from poorer health and development, and are more likely to die early than are those with coverage.**
• **Even one uninsured person in a family can put the financial stability and health of the whole family at risk.**
• **A community's high uninsured rate can adversely affect the overall health status of the community, its health care institutions and providers, and the access of its residents to certain services.**

---

[2]In this study, the focus is on people with no health insurance, such as "major medical" coverage for hospitalization and outpatient medical services, either for short or long periods. The Committee does not address *underinsurance*, that is, health plans that offer less than adequate coverage with excessive out-of-pocket payments, maximum benefit limits, or exclusion of specific services, such as mental health treatment. The problems of *underinsurance* are generally less severe than those of *uninsurance*, involve different policy issues, and require the collection of different types of information. See further discussion in Chapter 2.

• The estimated value across the population in healthy years of life gained by providing health insurance coverage is almost certainly greater than the additional costs of an "insured" level of services for those who now lack coverage.[3]

GUIDING THE DEBATE

In this report, the sixth and last in the series, the Committee presents its conclusions and recommendations, based on the findings of its previous five reports. It calls for action on the problems of uninsurance and hopes to stimulate informed discussion of the various proposals that have been put forth to extend coverage. *By "extend coverage" we mean having more people gain coverage who previously had had none and reducing the uninsured rate.* To guide future discussion, the Committee offers principles, supported by research, against which proposals for extending coverage can be assessed.

The Committee's review of clinical, epidemiological, and economic research for its earlier reports revealed certain features of health insurance that contribute to better health outcomes for those who have coverage. These insights into what accounts for the greater effectiveness of "insured" health care are reflected in the principles the Committee presents to guide policy makers and the public in analyzing proposals or developing new strategies. The Committee does not recommend or reject any specific proposal. Rather it demonstrates, through the use of the principles, how each of a wide range of proposals would improve the current situation.

ELIMINATING UNINSURANCE:
LESSONS FROM THE PAST AND PRESENT

Present-day efforts to reduce or eliminate uninsurance build on nearly a century of campaigns to bring about universal health insurance coverage. **Past campaigns have yielded both incremental changes and major reforms but not universal coverage, due to the challenges to major structural changes posed by American political arrangements and the lack of political leadership strong and sustained enough to forge a workable consensus on coverage legislation. In addition, the opposition of provider, insurer, and business groups with economic interests potentially adversely affected by specific reform proposals has blocked universal coverage even though many have agreed with the general need for reform.**

---

[3]An "insured" level of services reflects the current average benefits under Medicaid or private health insurance for those under age 65.

In the early 1900s, health insurance was seen initially as a type of social insurance, justified as a means of protecting workers' lost income when disabled or ill (Starr, 1982). By the 1930s it became a way to make health services more affordable for individuals and thus encourage utilization. Opposition to compulsory public insurance at the national level fed the development of private-sector nonprofit and commercial health coverage organized through the workplace. Between 1940 and 1960, the proportion of the general population with private health insurance grew from 9 percent to 68 percent (Bovbjerg et al., 1993).

Reform efforts to extend public coverage to retirees and the poor, two groups unlikely to purchase private coverage and likely to have difficulty paying for health care, met with success in 1965 with the enactment of Medicare and Medicaid as amendments to the Social Security Act. These two new programs introduced tens of millions of newly insured persons, and billions of new public dollars, into the health care system. Campaigns for universal coverage in the 1970s and 1990s have been shaped by the tensions between the goals of enrolling greater numbers of people and controlling health care expenditures.

Recent Federal Initiatives to Extend Coverage Have Not Closed the Coverage Gap

Finding: Federal incremental reforms over the past 20 years have made little progress in reducing overall uninsured rates nationally, although public program expansions have improved coverage for targeted previously uninsured groups. Federal reforms of employment-based insurance have not included provisions for assuring affordability and, thus, have had limited effect.

Finding: Extensions of program eligibility for one group of uninsured often affect the coverage status of other population groups indirectly, for example, when State Children's Health Insurance Program enrollment efforts identify children who are eligible for but not enrolled in Medicaid.

Finding: Public programs fall short of their coverage goals when not all eligible persons enroll. When outreach and enrollment are made a priority, coverage levels rise. Public coverage programs sometimes employ administrative barriers to enrollment to contend with inadequate or unstable funding during periods of economic stress within states.

Health insurance coverage rates nationally reached their high point in 1980, when approximately 15 percent of the general population under age 65 was uninsured (Bovbjerg et al., 1993). The percentage uninsured has not varied widely since then, but the number of uninsured people has grown substantially, to over

43 million, reflecting growth in the total population. Reforms since 1980 have made little progress in reducing the uninsured rate (Levit et al., 1992; Fronstin, 2002; Mills and Bhandari, 2003).

Since the mid-1980s, however, major federal initiatives to extend both public and private coverage, many modeled after successful state programs, have improved coverage rates among lower income children (in households earning less than 200 percent of poverty) and boosted the numbers of lower income persons with public coverage. Between 1984 and 1990, Congress gradually expanded Medicaid for pregnant women, infants, and young children, delinking coverage from welfare eligibility. These Medicaid expansions were followed in 1997 by the creation of the State Children's Health Insurance Program (SCHIP), a 10-year, $40 billion allotment in federal matching and capped grants in aid to the states. This program reduced the number of uninsured children, though more than half of the remaining uninsured children are eligible but not enrolled (Broaddus and Ku, 2000; Dubay et al., 2002a; Kenney et al., 2003).

Federal initiatives to extend employment-based coverage have targeted improved portability and continuity of coverage through the Consolidated Omnibus Budget Reconciliation Act of 1985 (COBRA), the Health Insurance Portability and Accountability Act of 1996 (HIPAA), and the Trade Act of 2002 (TA). All three statutes attempt to preserve coverage for specific categories of transitioning and unemployed workers and their families, yet the lack of authority or resources under COBRA and HIPAA to make insurance premiums affordable has seriously limited their usefulness and impact. It remains to be seen whether the subsidized tax credit to be given to displaced workers and retirees under the TA's authority will make premiums affordable enough to increase coverage among the approximately 260,000 eligible persons (Healthcare Leadership Council, 2003).

State and Local Initiatives to Extend Coverage

> Finding: The federal Employee Retirement Income Security Act of 1974 (ERISA) constrains the ability of states to mandate employment-based coverage, one strategy to extend private coverage within their boundaries.

> Finding: Although some states have made significant progress in reducing uninsurance, even the states that have led major coverage reforms have large and persisting uninsured populations.

> Finding: States do not have the fiscal resources to implement fully their existing public coverage programs and are further constrained from eliminating uninsurance within their boundaries by categorical limits on eligibility for federally supported public coverage programs.

Finding: Extensions of public or private coverage at the county level have focused on increasing coverage among targeted populations rather than the entire uninsured population locally. Despite the potential of local programs to fill targeted gaps, the lack of a reliable funding source limits their scope and effectiveness.

Historically some states have taken the lead in extending coverage, but state efforts alone have been insufficient to eliminate uninsurance within their boundaries and have had little impact on the overall, national uninsured rate. This report highlights five states—Hawaii, Massachusetts, Minnesota, Oregon, and Tennessee—that have invested significant funds since the mid-1980s to expand their public programs and in some cases have also regulated the small group and nongroup insurance markets to create more affordable options. In 1994, these states began using Medicaid Section 1115 waivers, without additional federal dollars, to broaden eligibility, with all but Tennessee folding in their own separate coverage programs for persons ineligible for Medicaid. Though all have made progress in extending coverage, each state still has significant numbers of uninsured people.

All states are limited by ERISA, which does not permit direct state regulation of coverage plans sponsored by private employers.[4] States may not tax employer-sponsored plans directly, require employers to offer coverage, or regulate what they do offer.

Addressing concerns about the substitution or crowding out of private coverage by new public programs has created administrative barriers to full enrollment of all eligible persons. The increasingly severe budget crises faced by the states beginning in 2001 have limited state reform and begun to erode coverage, although the prospect of losing federal revenue has motivated states to maintain much of their commitment to public coverage programs that receive federal matching funds (Smith et al., 2002; Boyd, 2003). State governments' capacity to finance health care and extend coverage tends to be weakest at times when demands for such support are likely to be highest, for example, during an economic recession. Nonetheless, the growing unmet need for health insurance in recent years has catalyzed reform efforts in many states (IOM, 2003a).

Many states designate their counties as the providers of last resort for the underserved and uninsured (IOM, 2003a). Across the nation, a handful of counties has experimented with innovative ways to improve access to care using insurance or an approach that resembles health insurance to reduce the impact of uninsurance on their communities. The Committee looked at the experiences of three urban counties that have led reform, Alameda County (CA), Hillsborough County (FL), and San Diego (CA). These counties have reformed the organization, financing, and delivery of local health services, combining outreach and enrollment activities

---

[4]In 1983, Hawaii received an exemption from ERISA, under the condition that the provisions of the state's employer mandate not be updated.

with new sources of revenue to support coverage. Serious financial constraints limit the scope and effectiveness of these programs and keep them from fully reaching their goals.

Despite gradual expansions of public programs at the federal, state, and local levels and isolated efforts around the country to move toward the goal of universal coverage, the lack of political consensus has prevented a substantial reduction in uninsurance in the United States. Laudable efforts have been hindered by a lack of resources. The state and county programs described here are noteworthy but atypical; individual state and local efforts to extend health insurance will not achieve universal coverage nationally. In some states the size of the uninsured population is overwhelming and many states lack the resources to extend coverage substantially. The circumscribed nature of past and present initiatives suggests that attempts to provide universal coverage without a substantial infusion of new federal funds are unrealistic. Recognition of the need to treat the elimination of uninsurance as a national responsibility, as well as a state and local one, is essential to comprehensive reform of coverage.

Conclusion: The persistence of uninsurance in the United States requires a national and coherent strategy aimed at covering the entire population. Federal leadership and federal dollars are necessary to eliminate uninsurance, although not necessarily federal administration or a uniform approach throughout the country. Universal health insurance coverage will only be achieved when the principle of universality is embodied in federal public policy.

A VISION OF UNIVERSAL COVERAGE

The Committee's previous reports detailed the negative effects on individuals' health, family stability, community health care institutions and access of residents, and the national economy associated with the existence of a large uninsured population. This report reviews a century of efforts aimed at reducing or eliminating uninsurance. This report also examines various approaches to providing health insurance because the Committee believes extending insurance coverage is a worthwhile and feasible endeavor. Imagine what the country would be like if everyone had coverage—people would be financially able to have a health problem checked, to seek preventive and primary care promptly, and to receive necessary, appropriate, and effective health services. Hospitals would be able to provide care without jeopardizing their operating budget and all families would have security in knowing that they had some protection against the prospect of medical bills undermining their financial stability or creditworthiness. The Committee believes that this picture could become reality and that it is an image worth pursuing because the costs of uninsurance to all of us—financial, societal, and in terms of health—are so great. The benefits of appropriate and timely health care are potentially even greater and can help motivate attaining this vision.

VISION STATEMENT

The Committee on the Consequences of Uninsurance envisions an approach to health insurance that will promote better overall health for individuals, families, communities, and the nation by providing financial access for everyone to necessary, appropriate, and effective health services.

PRINCIPLES TO GUIDE THE EXTENSION OF COVERAGE

The evidence reviewed and developed by the Committee in its first five reports contributes to this shared vision and the following five key principles. The first principle is the most basic and yet most important. The remaining four principles are not ranked by priority. Selected pieces of evidence are provided in the following discussion of the principles. (See the Committee's earlier reports, *Coverage Matters, Care Without Coverage, Health Insurance Is a Family Matter, A Shared Destiny*, and *Hidden Costs, Value Lost*, and Chapter 2 in the full report, *Insuring America's Health*, for more detailed discussions of the evidence.)

1. **Health care coverage should be universal.**
   • Everyone living in the United States should be covered by health insurance. Being uninsured can damage the health of individuals and families. Uninsured children and adults use medical and dental services less often than insured people and are less likely to receive routine preventive care (Newacheck et al., 1998b; McCormick et al., 2001; IOM, 2002b). They are also less likely to have a regular source of care than are insured people (Zuvekas and Weinick, 1999; Weinick et al., 2000). Insurance coverage is the best mechanism for gaining financial access to services that may produce better health.
   • Uninsured people are less likely to receive high-quality, professionally recommended care and medications, particularly for preventive services and chronic conditions (Beckles et al., 1998; Cooper-Patrick et al., 1999; Powell-Griner et al., 1999; Ayanian et al., 2000; Breen et al., 2001; Goldman et al., 2001).
   • Uninsured children risk abnormal long-term development if they do not receive routine care; uninsured adults have worse outcomes for chronic conditions such as diabetes, cardiovascular disease, end-stage renal disease, and HIV (Hadley, 2002; IOM, 2002a, b).
   • Uninsured adults have a 25 percent greater mortality risk than do insured adults, accounting for an estimated 18,000 excess deaths annually (Franks et al., 1993a; Sorlie et al., 1994; IOM, 2002a).

2. **Health care coverage should be continuous.**
   • Continuous coverage is more likely to lead to improved health outcomes;

breaks in coverage result in diminished health status (Lurie et al., 1984, 1986; Franks et al., 1993a; Sorlie et al., 1994; Baker et al., 2001).

• Achieving coverage well before the onset of an illness would likely lead to a better health outcome because the chance of early detection would be enhanced (Perkins et al., 2001).

• Interruptions in coverage interfere with therapeutic relationships, contribute to missed preventive services for children, and result in inadequate chronic care (Rodewald et al., 1997; Beckles et al., 1998; Burstin et al., 1998; Daumit et al., 1999, 2000; Hoffman et al., 2001).

3. Health care coverage should be affordable to individuals and families.

• The high cost of health insurance is the main reason people give for being uninsured (Hoffman and Schlobohm, 2000; IOM, 2001a). Nearly two-thirds of people with no coverage have incomes that are less than 200 percent of the federal poverty level (IOM, 2001a). Families in that income group have little leeway for health expenditures, making some form of financial assistance necessary for obtaining coverage (IOM, 2002b).

• Among families with no members insured during the entire year and incomes below the poverty level, more than a quarter paid out-of-pocket medical expenses that were more than 5 percent of income (Taylor et al., 2001).

4. The health insurance strategy should be affordable and sustainable for society.

• The Committee acknowledges that any health insurance strategy will likely face budgetary constraints on the benefits as well as on the administrative operations. Any major reform will need mechanisms to control the rate of growth in health care spending. There is no analytically derivable dollar amount of what society can afford; that will be determined through political and economic processes.

• The Committee believes that everyone should contribute financially to the national strategy through mechanisms such as taxes, premiums, and cost sharing because all members of society can expect to benefit from universal health insurance coverage.

• To help ensure affordability, the reform strategy should strive for efficiency and simplicity.

5. Health insurance should enhance health and well-being by promoting access to high-quality care that is effective, efficient, safe, timely, patient-centered, and equitable.

• Insurance should be designed to enhance the quality of the health care system as specified above and recommended by the IOM's Committee on Quality of Health Care in America (IOM, 2001b).

- A benefit package that includes preventive and screening services, outpatient prescription drugs, and specialty mental health care as well as outpatient and hospital services would enhance receipt of appropriate care (Huttin et al., 2000; IOM, 2002a).
- Variation in patient cost sharing could be used as an incentive for appropriate service use because it can influence patient behavior (Newhouse and The Insurance Experiment Group, 1993).

USING THE PRINCIPLES

The Committee's research on the problems related to uninsurance demonstrates conclusively that there are benefits for the nation and all its residents from eliminating uninsurance and ensuring coverage for everyone. Based on a review of past incremental and disjointed efforts to extend coverage, the limited progress made, and the remaining 43 million uninsured,

The Committee concludes that health insurance coverage for everyone in the United States requires major reform initiated as federal policy.

Achieving universal coverage across the country will require at a minimum federal policy direction and financial support. The new system would not necessarily be controlled wholly at the federal level or operated solely through a government agency. The Committee presents the preceding set of principles to be used in clarifying the public debate about approaches to extending coverage. The principles provide objectives against which to measure various proposals. The Committee does not endorse or reject any particular approach to solving the problem of uninsurance, but recognizes that there are many pathways to achieving its vision.

The Committee recommends that these principles be used to assess the merits of current proposals and to design future strategies for extending coverage to everyone.

To illustrate how the principles should be used to evaluate reform proposals, the Committee sketches four prototypes for major reform in a simplified format so that the main incentives are clear. It then assesses each prototype against each of the principles, highlighting the model's strengths and weaknesses. These models all include aspects of strategies under discussion in the public debate but are not detailed legislative proposals or specific strategies favored by particular politicians or advocacy groups. Brief outlines of the prototypes (discussed fully in Chapter 5 of *Insuring America's Health*) are as follows:

1. *Major public program extension and new tax credit:* No fundamental change in private insurance, Medicaid and SCHIP merged and expanded, Medicare extended to 55 year olds, a tax credit for moderate income individuals.

2. *Employer mandate, premium subsidy, and individual mandate*: Employers required to provide coverage and contribute to workers' premiums, subsidy for employers of low-wage workers, individuals required to accept employment-based insurance or obtain it privately, merged public program for those not covered at work.

3. *Individual mandate and tax credit*: Each person eligible for an advanceable, refundable tax credit and required to obtain coverage in the private market, Medicaid and SCHIP eliminated.

4. *Single payer*: Administered federally, everyone enrolled, single benefit package, global budget, no Medicaid, SCHIP, or Medicare.

Each model meets some principles better than others and each principle may be more fully achieved by one prototype than another. For example, the principle of universal coverage is more likely to be reached through any of the models with mandates than by the first prototype, which is entirely voluntary. Prototype 1 was included for completeness because it is an obvious approach currently under public consideration, although it would not achieve universality. The single payer model would most successfully eliminate gaps in coverage. The assessment of each model is fully discussed in Chapter 5 and summarized in Table ES.1.

The affordability to individuals and families of each prototype would depend on the size of the subsidies or tax credits and cost-sharing requirements, as well as eligibility levels for the public programs. The affordability and sustainability for society of each model would largely depend on the nature of cost controls in the system, sources of revenues, the amount of cost sharing, and the comprehensiveness of the benefit packages. Strong cost and utilization controls could affect access to services and health outcomes in ways yet to be determined. The Committee is mindful that defining a minimum benefit package for the uninsured would likely also affect some people who currently have a lesser insurance package, increasing their benefits and resulting in additional costs and probably increased access to services and drugs and improved health outcomes.

The potential of various models to enhance health through quality care would depend on the design of the benefit packages, the strength of the public programs, and effective consumer demand. There are some shortcomings of each model, but each prototype could come closer to achieving the Committee's vision and be ameliorated with further refinement, and elements of different models could be combined to promote particular principles. Most importantly, **each prototype could more nearly achieve each principle than does the current system.**

NEXT STEPS

The Committee recognizes that it will take some time to develop, adopt, and implement a program of universal coverage and that it will require additional public resources to finance insurance. It will not be quick or easy to implement the necessary reforms and it will be preferable to phase in the changes according to a fixed schedule. Implementation should aim for a minimum number of transi-

TABLE ES.1 Summary Assessment of Prototypes Based on Committee Principles

Principles	Status Quo	Prototype 1 Major Public Program Expansion and Tax Credit
Coverage should be universal	Not universal; *43 million uninsured*	*Would not achieve universality because voluntary,* but would reduce uninsured population
Coverage should be continuous	*Not continuous;* income, age, family, job, and health-related *gaps in coverage*	Family- and job-related *gaps in coverage*
Coverage should be affordable for individuals and families	*Private coverage unaffordable* to many moderate- and low-income persons	*More affordable than current system* for those with low or moderate income
Strategy should be affordable and sustainable for society	*Not affordable or sustainable for society;* uninsurance is growing; cost of poorer health and shorter lives is $65–$130 billion; some participants contribute; no limit on aggregate health expenditures or on tax expenditures—spending is higher than other countries; sustainability of current public programs depends on economy and political support	All participants contribute; *aggregate expenditures not controlled; new public expenditures for only the public program expansion and tax credit;* sustainability of public program depends on revenue sources and political support; size of credit depends on political support
Coverage should enhance health through high-quality care	*Quality of care* for the population *limited* because one in seven is uninsured	Opportunities to promote quality improvements *similar to current system*

Prototype 2	Prototype 3	Prototype 4
Employer Mandate, Premium Subsidy, and Individual Mandate	Individual Mandate and Tax Credit	Single Payer
Coverage likely to be high; depends on enforcement of mandates	*Depends on size of tax credit, enforcement,* and cost of individual insurance	*Likely to achieve universal coverage*
Brief gaps related to life and job transitions	*Minimal gaps*	*Continuous* until death or age 65
Yes for workers, assuming adequate employer premium assistance; *public program designed to be affordable* for all enrollees	Subsidy based only on income and family size leaves *older, less healthy, and those in expensive areas with less affordable coverage*	*Minimal cost sharing,* but could be problem for lowest income
All participants contribute; *basic package less costly than current employment coverage;* revenue from patients in public program; sustainability depends on revenue sources for employers' premium assistance and public program	No limit on aggregate health expenditures or on tax expenditure, though federal costs relatively predictable and controllable through size of credit; *sustainable through federal income tax base;* size of credit depends on political support	Nearly all participants contribute; *aggregate expenditures controllable,* utilization not directly or centrally controlled; *high cost to federal budget;* administrative savings; sustainability depends on revenue source and political support
Could design quality incentives in expanded public program and basic benefit package; current employer incentives for quality remain	*Similar incentives to current private insurance* system; consumer could choose quality plans	*Potentially yes;* depends on proper design

tional stages, each of which incorporates changes that are as coherent and simple as possible. Despite a long history of failed attempts to achieve insurance for everyone, the Committee believes that universal insurance coverage is an important and achievable goal for the country. Instead of considering the status quo as everyone's second choice when consensus on an approach to universal coverage fails to materialize, we should consider it the *last* choice. We cannot afford to ignore the problem of uninsurance.

The Committee recommends that the President and Congress develop a strategy to achieve universal insurance coverage and to establish a firm and explicit schedule to reach this goal by 2010.

The Committee recommends that, until universal coverage takes effect, the federal and state governments provide resources sufficient for Medicaid and SCHIP to cover all persons currently eligible and prevent the erosion of outreach efforts, eligibility, enrollment, and coverage.

The Committee is concerned that the current and growing economic pressures on state governments as well as at the federal level will have a negative impact on public programs and erode current coverage, making future coverage gains more difficult. Until everyone has financial access to health services through insurance, it is necessary to sustain current public coverage programs. It is also important to shore up the current capacity of health care institutions and providers who take a major responsibility for caring for the uninsured. Continuing support of service capacity, particularly in medically underserved areas, may be needed.

The Committee appreciates that making a national commitment to achieve universal insurance coverage will require strong, bipartisan political support as well as broad-based and deep public support. We all bear the costs of the current nonsystem that leaves tens of millions without health coverage. Doing nothing and maintaining the status quo with over 43 million uninsured Americans is expensive. The nation suffers losses due to ill health, impaired development, early deaths, and lost productivity. The lack of health insurance is a destabilizing factor in families and for health care institutions that serve uninsured patients. In fact, the presence of uninsurance creates insecurity for everyone, even those with health insurance today, because losing that coverage tomorrow is so easy. Universal insurance coverage will benefit all Americans, enhance the great promise of our health care system, and reinforce our values as a democratic society. **It is time for our nation to extend coverage to everyone.**

1

Introduction

The persistence of a large uninsured population in this country, regardless of the prevailing economic conditions, is remarkable. In 2000, when this three-year study of the consequences of uninsurance began, 39.4 million people under age 65 in the United States reported having no health insurance during the previous year.[1] The uninsured population had grown by more than 6 million during the 1990s, despite a decade of strong economic growth, when health care inflation slowed and health spending flattened at just over 13 percent of the *gross domestic product* (GDP) between 1992 and 2001.[2] Federal and state budgets had experienced surpluses, and states expanded their existing coverage programs and explored new opportunities to cover more of their uninsured populations. Yet at the height of this prosperous period, 1998–2000, the number of uninsured dropped by less than a million; see Figure 1.1. In 2000, the uninsured rate began to grow once more. Despite fluctuations in economic and demographic trends, which can affect the numbers and percentage of the population insured, a large uninsured population has persisted over the past few decades.

---

[1]The estimate of 39.4 million uninsured is based on the Census Bureau's March Current Population Survey (CPS) as are all annual estimates of the uninsured population of the United States presented in this report, unless otherwise noted. See Chapter 2 and Appendix A for a more detailed discussion of various measures of the uninsured rate and length of time people are uninsured, why they are uninsured, and characteristics of the uninsured.

[2]Italicized technical terms are defined in the glossary (Appendix B).

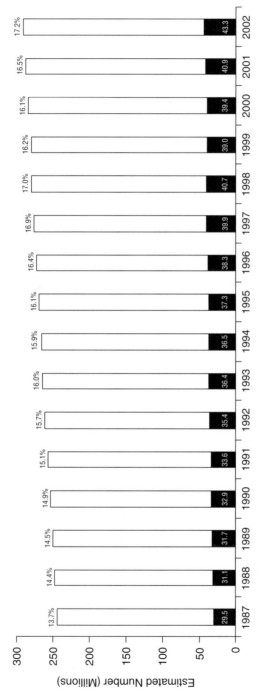

FIGURE 1.1 Uninsured persons under age 65, number and proportion of general population under age 65, 1987–2002.
NOTE: Estimates for 2000, 2001, and 2002 use Census 2000-based weights.
SOURCES: Fronstin, 2002; Mills and Bhandari, 2003.

Now, the uninsured population continues to increase in number, and the uninsured rate is expected to worsen in the continuing weak economy (Fronstin, 2002). Over 43 million people were reported uninsured in 2002, representing 17.2 percent of the population under the age of 65 (Mills and Bhandari, 2003).[3] Unemployment is up now, state budgets are experiencing increased demands for services, state revenues are less than had been anticipated, and many states have significant budget shortfalls (National Governors Association, 2003; Rowland, 2003; U.S. Bureau of Labor Statistics, 2003a). The federal budget has returned to a deficit position as well. Health costs and health insurance premiums are again increasing faster than general inflation and more quickly than family and business incomes (Heffler et al., 2003; U.S. Bureau of Labor Statistics, 2003b). Many states are proposing or implementing cost containment measures for public coverage programs, although few have yet to cut eligibility substantially or covered services for their Medicaid and State Children's Health Insurance Programs (SCHIP) and some are pursuing significant extensions of coverage as a means to reduce uncompensated care costs (Holahan et al., 2003d; Ross and Cox, 2003; Smith et al., 2003).

The problem of uninsurance has been growing in urgency, not just because of the economy and increasing numbers of uninsured Americans. Insurance is so important now because the effectiveness of medical interventions, particularly medical technologies and pharmaceuticals, continues to increase, improving health and longevity (Cutler and Richardson, 1997; Murphy and Topel, 1999; Heidenreich and McClellan, 2003). Without insurance, people have less access to these new services and drugs. Thus, the gap between insured and uninsured people widens and raises questions of equity. This disparity in accesss to health care violates generally accepted American values of equal consideration and equal opportunity (IOM, 2003b).

The failure of many attempts throughout the past century to extend health insurance coverage to everyone is a notable feature of health care in the United States. The lack of universal health insurance coverage places this nation along with Mexico and Turkey as the only ones among the developed countries around the globe with substantial uninsured populations (OECD, 2002). It is time to rethink the nation's approach to financing access to health care for its population.

PURPOSE OF THE PROJECT AND THIS REPORT

In 2000, the Institute of Medicine (IOM) formed the Committee on the Consequences of Uninsurance to examine the evidence concerning the lack of health insurance for those without coverage, for their families, for their commu-

---

[3]Unless otherwise stated, this report will focus on the population under age 65 because the federal Medicare program provides nearly universal coverage for people at and above that age.

nities, and for this country as a whole. Most often, an IOM study is self-contained in a single report that lays out the evidence leading to the Committee's findings and conclusions and then proceeds to make recommendations. This project is unusual in that it was designed to produce six reports during the course of the three-year study that examine the issue of uninsurance critically and methodically from several different perspectives. The first five reports present evidence, findings, and conclusions on their given topics (see following descriptions of each). As planned from the outset, the Committee has withheld most of its recommendations until it fully examined the issue. Therefore, this sixth and final report draws on the findings of the previous five reports, as well as an examination of selected historical efforts and federal, state, and local programs that were designed to extend coverage. *The Committee uses the term "extend coverage" to mean having more people gain coverage who previously had had none and reducing the uninsured rate.* That extension of coverage could be achieved through either expansion of existing insurance programs or creation of new mechanisms.

The findings from the six reports as a whole have convinced the Committee that uninsurance is a critical problem for the United States that can and should be eliminated. The Committee believes that leaving over 43 million Americans uninsured is costly to the country and should no longer be tolerated.

The intent in this final report is to present principles based on the Committee's previous research, apply them to potential strategies to extend coverage and eliminate uninsurance, and make a strong case for taking action now. Although the report examines a wide range of approaches that have been proposed to extend coverage, it does not recommend a particular proposal. Rather, it presents principles and recommendations to guide the public, policy makers, and elected officials in crafting effective and achievable solutions. This report also provides examples of how to apply the principles to assess the strengths and weaknesses of various strategies to extend coverage.

FINDINGS AND CONCLUSIONS FROM PREVIOUS COMMITTEE REPORTS

The Committee's first five reports identify the many consequences for the country of maintaining such a large uninsured population:

- *Coverage Matters: Insurance and Health Care* (IOM, 2001a) provides an overview of how health insurance works in America, and describes the socioeconomic and demographic characteristics of uninsured populations. It also sets out a conceptual framework for thinking about uninsurance; this framework has guided the analyses in all the following reports (see Figure 1.2 below).
- *Care Without Coverage: Too Little, Too Late* (IOM, 2002a) assesses the clinical research concerning health consequences for uninsured adults, including over-

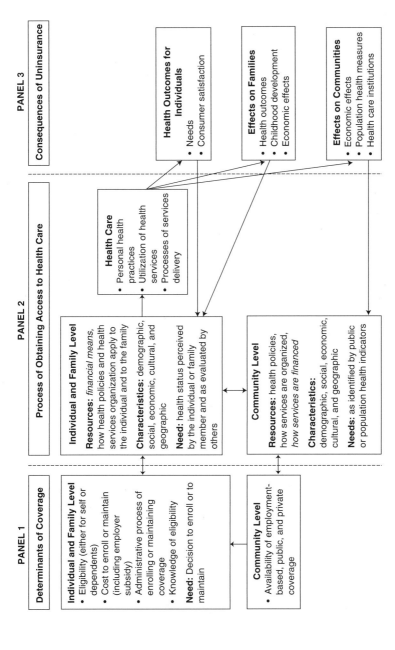

FIGURE 1.2 A conceptual framework for evaluating the consequences of uninsurance—a cascade of effects.
NOTE: Italics indicate terms that include direct measures of health insurance coverage.
SOURCE: IOM, 2001a.

all health status, the incidence of specific diseases, avoidable hospitalizations, the *quality of care* received, preventable morbidity, and premature mortality.

• *Health Insurance Is a Family Matter* (IOM, 2002b) examines similar health effects for children and pregnant women. In addition, it expands the focus beyond the individual to include the effects of one or more uninsured family members on others in the family, including those with insurance, and on the family as a unit.

• *A Shared Destiny: Community Effects of Uninsurance* (IOM, 2003a) looks at wider "spillover" effects of uninsurance on the local community, insured as well as uninsured residents, and specifically on its health care providers.

• *Hidden Costs, Value Lost: Uninsurance in America* (IOM, 2003b) details the costs to the country of sustaining such a large uninsured population. Many of the costs identified in the earlier reports are quantified. The costs of additional health care services likely to be used by those who are now uninsured, if they were to gain coverage, are also calculated.

The Committee concludes that allowing a sizable uninsured population to persist has serious negative consequences for individuals, families, communities, and the entire nation.

Collectively, these five reports show that current insurance mechanisms have not eliminated the large, persistent uninsured population and indeed are not structured to do so. The current system relies on an assortment of private and public sources to provide coverage, each of which meets the needs of some people, while leaving millions uncovered. Instead of approaching the problem in tentative incremental steps, the Committee believes that citizens and policy makers should begin by setting as an explicit goal that the health insurance system should include everyone, then determine the private and public policies and actions necessary to achieve that end, and enact and implement those policies.

The Committee concludes that major, comprehensive reform of the health insurance system, rather than expansion of the "safety net," is essential.

The "safety net" loosely refers to health care facilities and programs that disproportionately serve needy and uninsured people. If financial access to health care services were assured, people would be able to choose among providers in their community and not be dependent upon safety-net institutions, as uninsured people are now. Also, the availability of payments from insurers could strengthen the financial stability of those providers and institutions, which are stressed by the current economy and growing demands for services (IOM, 2003a; KCMU, 2003a). Safety-net services, institutions, and accommodating providers vary widely from state to state and area to area, have ill-defined responsibilities, are inadequate to meet current needs of the uninsured, and are unlikely to meet future needs (Lewin and Altman, 2000; Hadley, 2002; IOM, 2003a).

Strengthening safety-net services would not be an adequate alternative to expanding health insurance coverage. For example, federally supported primary care clinics, including community health centers, have a heavy case load of uninsured clients but serve only 6.5 to 10 percent of the total uninsured population. Most uninsured people do not live near a center (Cunningham and Tu, 1997; IOM, 2003a). Persons receiving primary care in such centers often have difficulty obtaining specialty, diagnostic, and behavioral health services for which they are referred (Gusmano et al., 2002). An analysis of 13 states shows that access for uninsured lower income adults varies depending on local services capacity. However, even more striking in this analysis are the large gaps in access and use between the insured and uninsured populations in each state, regardless of the extent of local safety-net services (Holahan and Spillman, 2002). An analysis of racial disparities in access to care, based on national data from the Community Tracking Study (1996–1997 and 1998–1999), showed that lack of insurance is a significant barrier to access and more important than the supply of medical providers and services in the community (Hargraves and Hadley, 2003). Thus, the Committee has concentrated on insurance-based financing mechanisms, not necessarily tied to one provider or facility, to facilitate access to care rather than on programs that might increase the availability of certain services in selected geographic areas.

The Committee's definitions of health insurance and uninsured status are consistent with those adopted in its previous reports. Health insurance is defined by the Committee as financial coverage for basic hospital and ambulatory care services, whether provided through employment-based indemnity, service-benefit, or managed care plans; individually purchased health insurance policies; public programs such as Medicare (which covers virtually all persons 65 years of age and older), Medicaid, and the SCHIP; or other state-sponsored coverage for specified populations. *Uninsured* refers to persons without *any* form of public or private coverage for hospital and outpatient care, for any given length of time. In large part this operational definition reflects that used in virtually all studies that attempt to discern and measure the impact of coverage status on health and other individual and community outcomes. Although length of time without coverage almost certainly will make a difference, the information typically available about individual health insurance status (at baseline or inception of a study) tends to obscure differences between insured and uninsured populations and thus likely underestimates the negative effects of being uninsured.

Throughout its series of reports, the Committee has not attempted to address the condition of *underinsurance*, by which is meant individuals or families whose health insurance policy or benefits plan offers less than adequate coverage. The problems faced by the underinsured are in some respects similar to those faced by the uninsured, although they are generally less severe (IOM, 2002a, b). *Unin*surance and *under*insurance involve some distinctly different policy issues and the strategies for addressing them may differ. Throughout these reports, the Committee's main focus has been on persons with *no* health insurance and thus no assistance in paying for health care beyond what is available through charity and safety-net arrangements.

A COMPARISON OF THE UNITED STATES AND OTHER DEVELOPED COUNTRIES

Having insurance improves access to health services, and access to health care is associated with better health among the uninsured. (See Figure 1.2, the conceptual framework that has guided this project.) The health care provided in America's best medical centers is world renowned; many people come from abroad to benefit from the high-quality care available in this country. Tens of millions of Americans, however, are uninsured and do not receive the services they need (IOM, 2002a, b).

In the United States, health insurance has evolved from a mechanism to protect against only infrequent and serious health events and expenses to one that also finances routine health care and encourages the use of preventive services (IOM, 2001a). In addition to lowering financial barriers to care, health insurance improves the receipt of appropriate care by facilitating the use of a regular source of care or primary care provider. Coverage is an important determinant of obtaining and maintaining an ongoing relationship with a health care provider (IOM, 2001a; Holahan and Spillman, 2002). Even if uninsured persons receive primary care, referrals to specialists, ancillary diagnostic and treatment services, and medications are more difficult to obtain without coverage (Fairbrother et al., 2002). Both continuity of care and continuity of insurance coverage are important; breaks in coverage can disrupt care relationships to the detriment of high-quality health care. Being uninsured for longer periods of time can be expected to have larger negative effects on utilization of services (and consequently on health) than being uninsured for shorter periods (IOM, 2002a). The 43 million Americans who lack health insurance coverage for a year or more are more likely to suffer worse health and die sooner than Americans with health insurance (IOM, 2002a, b).

A comparison of the health care system in the United States and the average health of the U.S. population with that found in other countries highlights the reason why Americans should be dissatisfied with the status quo. Although the health care system in this country has accomplished a great deal, it can do much better in improving the quality of health services and the health of its population. Lowering financial barriers to needed health services is one important improvement to achieve this goal.

Table 1.1 includes health system and health status indicators of the United States and several other developed, high-income countries.[4] Several conclusions can be drawn from this table and the comparative international literature reviewed:

1. *The United States ranks the highest in health care spending per capita and as a percentage of GDP.* In 2000, the United States spent 13 percent of its GDP and

---

[4]Much of these comparative data are based on the total population, including persons over age 65.

TABLE 1.1 Health Care System Indicators in Selected Countries, 1997–2000

	1	2	3	4	5
Country	Total Health Spending as a Percent of GDP 2000	Health Spending Per Capita in U.S. Dollars 2000[a]	Infant Mortality Rate, Deaths per 1,000 Live Births 2000	Disability-Adjusted Life Expectancy in Years 1997–1999	% Total Population Publicly Covered 2000
United States	**13.0**	**4,631**	**6.9**	**70.0**	**86[b]**
Australia	8.3	2,211	5.2	73.2	100
Canada	9.1	2,535	5.3	72.0	100
Denmark	8.3	2,420	5.3	69.4	100[c]
Finland	6.6	1,664	3.8	70.5	100
France	9.5	2,349	4.6	73.1	99.8
Germany	10.6	2,748	4.4	70.4	92.2[d]
Italy	8.1	2,032	4.5	72.7	100
Japan	7.8	2,012	3.2	74.5	100
Luxembourg	NA	NA	5.1	71.1	100[d]
Norway	7.8	2,362	3.8	71.7	100
Sweden	NA	NA	3.4	73.0	100
Switzerland	10.7	3,222	4.9	72.5	100
United Kingdom	7.3	1,762	5.6	71.7	100

NOTES:

[a]Adjusted for cost-of-living differences, purchasing power parities.

[b]86 percent of total population was insured; 24 percent of total population was publicly covered in 2000 (Mills, 2001).

[c]1999 data.

[d]1997 data; Germany's insured rate is close to 99 percent including primary private insurance (Personal communication, Jeremy Hurst, OECD, September 11, 2003).

SOURCES: (Columns 1,2,3,5: OECD, 2002; column 4: WHO, 2000).

$4,631 per capita on health care (Table 1.1, columns 1 and 2) (OECD, 2002). This spending far surpassed the next most expensive health care systems, those of Switzerland (10.7 percent of GDP) and Germany (10.6 percent of GDP). The per capita amount spent in the United States is more than twice that of most of the other countries of similar economic standing. While the U.S. spends substantially more than the other countries, its measures of use of services, such as physician visits and hospital days per capita, are below the Organization for Economic Cooperation and Development (OECD) median (Anderson et al., 2003). The implication is that the prices of those services are higher in the U.S. (Anderson et al., 2003).

2. *The health care system in the United States is deemed to be the most responsive in the world* to nonhealth aspects of care, such as respect for the individual, protection of confidentiality, opportunity to participate in choices of treatments and providers, provision of prompt attention, and clean surroundings (WHO, 2000).[5] The OECD, in a recent assessment of the performance of the U.S. health care system, similarly found that it is very responsive to consumer preferences. For example, there is virtually no waiting time for elective procedures in the United States, unlike many OECD member countries and most Americans are highly satisfied with the care they receive (Docteur et al., 2003).

3. *Comparative international surveys document the high availability of medical technology in the United States and the fact that it is intensively used* (Docteur et al., 2003). For example, the United States was quicker to adopt and diffuse new technologies involved with care of heart attack patients than most of the 17 other developed countries studied (TECH Research Network, 2001). The number of coronary angioplasties in the United States per 100,000 population is more than two times that in Germany and even further ahead of Australia, Canada, New Zealand, and England. While the rates are not adjusted for disease prevalence, the large difference in rates suggests different patterns of treatment and diffusion of new treatments and technologies (Anderson et al., 2003). Compared with Australia, Canada, France, Germany, Japan, New Zealand, and the United Kingdom, the United States is second only to Japan in the availability of magnetic resonance imaging units: 23.2 in Japan versus 8.1 units in the United States per one million population. The United States has 14 computed tomography scanners per million persons, compared with Japan (84), Australia (21), Germany (17), and the OECD median (12) (Anderson et al., 2002).

4. *Although the United States ranks highest in health care spending (in total and as a percentage of GDP) and ranks high in the availability of medical technology, this spending has not produced comparably high measures of health status.* The health of Americans

---

[5]It should be noted that some of the World Health Organization rankings, while innovative, have been controversial. For the responsiveness ranking, the data were gathered from nearly 2000 key informants in 35 countries and the distribution of responsiveness for the remaining countries (156) was estimated using indirect techniques (WHO, 2000; Musgrove, 2003).

consistently ranks poorly relative to that of residents of other industrialized nations. Certainly the health status of a population reflects more than just medical care and the heterogeneity of the U.S. population distinguishes it from many other developed countries. Nonetheless, international comparisons provide a useful perspective on our own society and indicate areas for improvement.

A comparison of 13 countries based on 16 health indicators conducted by Barbara Starfield (2000) determined the United States ranked among the worst, on average twelfth. The countries included in the study were, in order from the top ranked (best health status) to the lowest, as follows: Japan, Sweden, Canada, France, Australia, Spain, Finland, the Netherlands, United Kingdom, Denmark, Belgium, United States, and Germany. The United States came in last for three indicators (low birth weight; neonatal mortality and infant mortality overall; years of potential life lost), even after excluding external causes such as motor vehicle collisions and violence. Also, OECD comparisons ranked the United States twenty-fifth in male life expectancy and nineteenth in female life expectancy out of 29 developed countries.

Infant mortality rates and life expectancy, and also disability-adjusted life expectancy (DALE), are among the most commonly used measures of population health. They are widely considered valid indicators of the overall effectiveness of the health care system, although many other factors also affect the health of a population.[6] As of 2000, the infant mortality rate in the United States was 6.9 infant deaths per 1,000 live births (OECD, 2002). Although this number represented a historic low for the United States, our infant mortality rate is nonetheless the highest among the listed countries (see Table 1.1, column 3). Even if one considers the U.S. infant mortality rate (5.7) for white infants only, whose mothers generally have a higher social and economic status than nonwhite mothers, it is still a higher rate than all the other countries. The 2000 infant mortality rate for black infants in the United States (14.1 deaths per 1,000 live births) was more than twice the white rate of 5.7 (National Center for Health Statistics, 2002).

Starfield found that, among the 13 countries she studied, the United States came in eleventh for life expectancy of females at age 1 and twelfth for males at age 1. Table 1.1, (column 4), shows that the United States has a DALE of 70 years. Of those countries listed in Table 1.1, only Denmark had a lower DALE, 69.4 years.

5. The United States is among the few industrialized nations in the world that *does not guarantee access* to health care for its population (see Table 1.1, column 5). Of 30 industrialized countries included in OECD health data, only Mexico and Turkey have higher uninsured rates. Nearly all the OECD countries provide public insurance for 99 to 100 percent of their population; Germany has substantially higher coverage than the 92.2 percent publicly covered, when primary private health insurance is included (OECD, 2002; personal communication,

---

[6]Disability-adjusted life expectancy is the number of healthy years of life that can be expected on average in a given population (WHO, 2000).

Jeremy Hurst, OECD, September 11, 2003). In contrast, only 86 percent of the U.S. population had health insurance in 2000, 24 percent covered by public programs (Mills, 2001).

The way that health care is organized and delivered in the United States and the limited access of uninsured persons contribute to our country's relatively low-ranking health indicators, despite high levels of spending. The OECD assessment of the United States concluded that "Incomplete insurance coverage and delayed access to care adversely affect population health outcomes and possibly economic performance" (Docteur et al., 2003, p.41). The IOM Committee on Assuring the Health of the Public in the 21st Century also found that the health of the American population is compromised by the lack of insurance for so many (IOM, 2003c). These findings are clearly consistent with the findings of the first five reports in this project on uninsurance. The large disparities in access to care and health outcomes experienced between the insured and the 15 percent of the total population that is uninsured in the United States may explain, in part, the low national rankings despite high spending.

HEALTH CARE REFORM AND HEALTH INSURANCE REFORM

This report distinguishes between the *health care delivery system* and the *health insurance system*. The primary focus of this project is on health insurance.[7] Reform of the health care delivery system is beyond the scope of this Committee's work, although other IOM Committees have identified serious problems with the system and made recommendations for reform. This report recognizes the work of those IOM Committees and the problems they have identified, noting the inter-relatedness of delivery system reform with strategies to reform health insurance (Field et al, 1993; Edmunds and Coye, 1998; Smedley and Syme, 2000; IOM, 2001b, 2003c; Corrigan et al., 2003; Smedley et al., 2002). Box 1.1 presents some findings from key IOM reports, listed chronologically by the date of their release.

Reform of the health care delivery system requires attention to issues such as cost control mechanisms, quality improvement, health workforce training, medi-

---

[7]In this country, neither health care nor health insurance can be characterized as a system and the Committee uses the word "system" with some hesitation. Our previous research makes it clear that health insurance in this country more closely resembles a hodgepodge or a patchwork quilt than an organized system. There are numerous ad hoc arrangements that vary from state to state, often leaving big gaps in coverage. Public coverage programs are targeted to specific subsets of the population; regulation of private insurance varies substantially by state and is constrained by federal and state laws; private employment-based coverage depends on the types of businesses in the area as well as economic conditions; and no single agency or person has responsibility for pulling together the pieces to ensure coverage for the whole population. Nonetheless, for convenience this report will use the term "health insurance system" when it refers broadly to the issues, players, and programs mentioned above that relate to financial access to care.

cal liability compensation systems, and implementation of information technology systems to promote more effective care patterns and administrative procedures. After careful examination, the IOM Committee on Quality of Health Care in America concluded that "The American health care delivery system is in need of fundamental change" and systemwide reform (IOM, 2001b). Changes in all these areas could contribute to better and more efficient health care for all and to improved opportunities for covering those without health insurance. The quality and cost of health care certainly can be affected by the health insurance system, and the reverse is also true. The Committee on the Consequences of Uninsurance, however, did not undertake the scope of research necessary to recommend reform of the entire care delivery system. It has focused on the effect of financial access to that system through health insurance. **This Committee urges that extension of health coverage not be delayed until the whole health care delivery system is reformed first, nor should the transformation of care delivery be delayed until all Americans are insured.** Reform of both the health care delivery system and the insurance system should move ahead expeditiously and consider the long-range goals of each as well as the overall evolution of health care.

ORGANIZATION OF THIS REPORT

The next chapter of this report presents the key findings and conclusions from all five of this Committee's previous reports in a systematic way to show the basis for its recommendations in this report. Because the earlier reports include all the research supporting each finding, only the most relevant studies are cited in this chapter.

The third chapter provides a historical overview of selected efforts during the past century to provide comprehensive coverage to the whole population or to the uninsured segment of it. It also examines several different approaches to extending health insurance coverage that have been implemented over the past 15 years, including examples from federal, state, and local programs in the public and private sectors.

Chapter 4 presents the Committee's guiding principles for reforming the health insurance system. The Committee recognizes as important certain evidence-based principles that describe characteristics of an effective health insurance system, regardless of its particular structure. The principles can be used to examine current proposals to extend health insurance coverage and to help develop new approaches that would combine the best of existing ideas or break new ground.

In Chapter 5 the Committee sketches several prototypical approaches to fundamental reform that vary quite dramatically in the means they propose to use to move toward universal coverage. They are drawn from the broad range of insurance extension options that have been put forth by various interest groups, policy analysts, and political groups of all persuasions. The wide range of these proposals demonstrates that there are potentially many pathways to achieving

BOX 1.1
Other Institute of Medicine Reports

1. The Committee on Assessing Health Care Reform Proposals concluded in *Assessing Health Care Reform* that improved access and health status required more than just financial access. It should include:

- broad public health and health education initiatives;
- efforts to structure services, systems, and financing to more effectively reach special populations;
- expanded access to primary and preventive services;
- clinical and health services research; and
- programs of quality assurance (Field et al., 1993).

2. The Committee on Children, Health Insurance, and Access to Care, in *America's Children*, evaluated evidence about the link between coverage and access to health care for children, with particular attention to the availability of care for uninsured and underserved children. It concluded that all children should have health insurance. In addition, it found a lack of affordable health insurance products that address the specific needs of children, including those with chronic or special needs, and it found that inadequate efforts for outreach and enrollment procedures and insufficient coordination efforts of public programs hinder enrollment (Edmunds and Coye, 1998).

3. The Committee on Capitalizing on Social Science and Behavioral Research to Improve the Public's Health, in *Promoting Health*, focused on social and behavioral factors, such as smoking, diet, alcohol use, sedentary life style, and accidents, which influence the health and disease of the American population. It recommended:

- a better balance between the clinical approach to disease and social and behavioral determinants of disease, injury, and disability; and
- interventions that link multiple levels—individual, interpersonal, institutional, community, and policy levels (Smedley and Syme, 2000).

4. The Committee on Quality of Health Care in America, in *Crossing the Quality Chasm*, recommended:

- redesigning health care processes to establish continuous healing relationships, evidence-based decision making, patient safety, the reduction of waste in the health system, and cooperation among clinicians;
- building an information infrastructure to support care delivery; and

fundamental reform. To show how the principles can be used, they are applied to the prototypes we present so that the strengths and limitations of each approach are revealed.

In the sixth and last chapter, the Committee presents its recommendations concerning health insurance. They are based on the findings in Chapter 3 concerning coverage extensions and those enumerated in Chapter 2, and on the

- structuring payment systems to promote quality care, which should be safe, effective, patient-centered, timely, efficient, and equitable (IOM, 2001b).

5. The Committee on Rapid Advance Demonstration Projects: Health Care Finance and Delivery Systems, in *Fostering Rapid Advances in Health Care*, highlighted problems of the health care delivery system for coverage of the uninsured, chronic care, primary care, information and communications technology infrastructure, and medical liability that could be ameliorated by the establishment of multiple demonstrations to test reform options. It included recommendations that the federal government commit funds for 10 years for demonstrations in three to five states to extend stable, affordable coverage through the use of tax credits, or eligibility expansions of Medicaid and SCHIP, or a combination approach (Corrigan et al., 2003).

6. The Committee on Understanding and Eliminating Racial and Ethnic Disparities in Health Care, in *Unequal Treatment*, recommended a comprehensive, multilevel strategy to eliminate disparities, including:

- strengthening of patient-provider relationships in publicly funded health plans;
- using clinical, evidence-based guidelines to promote consistency and equity of care;
- providing economic incentives for physician practices to reduce communications barriers;
- using the payment systems to ensure an adequate supply of services to minority patients; and
- employing multidisciplinary treatment and preventive care teams (Smedley et al., 2002).

7. The Committee on Assuring the Health of the Public in the 21st Century, in *The Future of Public Health in the 21st Century*, described numerous public health problems, including:

- an inadequate public health infrastructure;
- lack of knowledge about the determinants of population health; and
- the mismatch between health care spending and health outcomes.

This Committee concluded that adequate population health cannot be achieved if comprehensive and affordable health care is not available to everyone in the United States (IOM, 2003c).

findings and conclusions in the Committee's previous five reports. The recommendations also articulate fundamental shared values across the diverse Committee membership. The Committee's intention is that this report, and indeed the whole project, should both encourage and inform public debates about the uninsured and make those debates accessible to a wide range of Americans.

2

Lessons from Previous Reports

In this chapter the Committee reviews findings from its five previous reports that document the health and financial repercussions of being uninsured for individuals, families, communities, and the nation.[1] The chapter is structured as a series of questions whose answers are fundamental to understanding why it is necessary to redesign our country's overall approach to health insurance coverage.

- The first section examines the scope of uninsurance and current coverage patterns by identifying how many people lack insurance, their basic economic and demographic characteristics, the ways people obtain and lose coverage, current barriers to coverage, and the potential for growth in the uninsured population in the near future.
- The second section reports findings on how the lack of coverage affects access to and timely use of appropriate health care services, and adverse health outcomes for children and adults without health insurance.
- The third section reviews family and community effects of uninsurance: financial repercussions for family budgets, the extent of uncompensated health care, and potential impacts of large uninsured populations on community access to care and on the economic and physical health of communities.
- The fourth section outlines available evidence and projections of the current cost to the nation of uninsurance by looking at *out-of-pocket* expenditures of families, the cost of uncompensated care, an estimate of the value of life and health

---

[1]This chapter summarizes material presented in earlier reports. Evidence cited in the Committee's previous reports is updated where newer data are available.

lost due to uninsurance, and the potential for offsetting the cost of extended coverage.[2]

• The fifth section of this chapter looks at how the structure of insurance can affect health care usage and health outcomes, for example, how employment-based insurance, differing eligibility rules for public coverage for persons within the same family, and the cost and availability of individual health insurance policies can result in coverage gaps.

• The chapter concludes with a statement of the Committee's perspective on health insurance in America.

UNDERSTANDING THE SCOPE OF UNINSURANCE AND SOURCES OF COVERAGE

Americans are often unaware of the characteristics of people who lack health insurance (IOM, 2001a). More than 80 percent of uninsured children and adults under the age of 65 live in working families and about the same percentage are U.S. citizens (Hoffman and Wang, 2003). People may lack coverage regardless of age, education, or state of residence. Nearly two-thirds of all uninsured persons are members of lower income families (earning less than 200 percent of the *federal poverty level*, or FPL), however.

In this section the Committee reviews how many people are uninsured, how coverage is gained or lost, and the pathways and barriers to health coverage. Several alternative economic scenarios are also described, suggesting that without a fundamental change in national policy, the uninsured population is projected to continue growing.

How Many People Lack Health Insurance and Who Are They?

Estimates of the number of uninsured Americans depend on how uninsurance is measured. Increasingly, the lack of health insurance is understood as a condition for which virtually all Americans are to some extent at risk over the course of their lives, particularly at transitional points such as the age of majority or the loss of student status, rather than as a fixed characteristic of a well-defined segment of the population. Not all people, however, are equally at risk of being uninsured nor are all spells of uninsurance of equal length.

During 2002, the Current Population Survey (CPS), conducted annually by the Census Bureau, showed that approximately 43.6 million people in the United States reported being without health insurance coverage for the entire year (Mills and Bhandari, 2003).[3] Some analysts believe that the CPS estimate is closer to a

---

[2]Italicized terms are defined in the glossary (Appendix B).

[3]The Committee's series of reports has relied on the CPS annual estimates of the number of uninsured persons in the United States. See Appendix A for a discussion of the features and limitations of various national surveys measuring insurance status.

point-in-time count of uninsured Americans than it is of those uninsured for an entire year. In 2000 the CPS added a verification question to improve the accuracy of its estimates, which reduced the estimate of the full-year uninsured population, although the CPS still probably overestimates full-year uninsurance. The CPS, however, provides the most consistent data on health insurance coverage over time and is the most widely used source of information on coverage. The Committee has used this historical series as its basic data set throughout the study for these reasons.

Other data sets, the Survey of Income and Program Participation (SIPP) and the Medical Expenditure Panel Survey (MEPS), provide more precise information on length of time without coverage. An analysis of MEPS data found that one out of every three Americans under age 65, 80.2 million people, lacked health insurance for at least one month during a two-year period, while 23.5 million persons under age 65 were uninsured *throughout* that period (1996-1997), and 31.6 million were uninsured throughout 1996 (Short, 2001). A recent Congressional Budget Office publication compared SIPP and MEPS, which reported 21 and 31 million persons under age 65, respectively, who were uninsured for the entire year 1998 (CBO, 2003). The latest SIPP reports that, over the 48-month period calendar years 1996 through 1999, the overall median spell without health insurance lasted just under six months (Bhandari and Mills, 2003). Two separate analyses of MEPS (using some combination of data for 1996, 1997, and 1998) found that the average monthly count of uninsured persons for at least a one-year period is 45 million (Short, 2001; Hadley and Holahan, 2003a). People with low family income tend to remain uninsured for longer periods of time than those with incomes above the poverty level (McBride, 1997).

Socioeconomic and demographic indicators help characterize those who go without health insurance and identify who is most likely to go without insurance. Full-time, full-year employment offers families the best chances of acquiring and keeping health insurance, as does an annual income of greater than 200 percent of FPL.[4] While white, non-Hispanic people make up about half of the uninsured, minority group members have a higher risk of being uninsured. African Americans are nearly twice as likely as non-Hispanic whites to be uninsured, and Latinos are more than three times as likely as non-Hispanic whites to lack

---

[4]In 2003, 200 percent of FPL is $36,800 for a family of four (DHHS, 2003). (See Appendix A, Table A.1.) In this report, family income levels are defined as follows:

- Low income: an annual income of less than 100 percent of FPL, which is established on a yearly basis for different types of family groups that comprise a given household, for example, one adult, or one adult and two children;
- Lower income: an annual income of less than 200 percent of FPL; and
- Moderate income: an annual income of between 200 and 400 percent of FPL for a given family group.

coverage. Although most uninsured persons under age 65 are U.S. citizens (79 percent), foreign-born, noncitizen residents are more likely than citizens to be uninsured (Hoffman and Wang, 2003). The uninsured rate declines with the length of time foreign-born persons are in the United States: 42 percent of noncitizens living in the United States for more than 5 years are uninsured, compared with 50 percent of noncitizens in the country for less than 5 years (Hoffman and Wang, 2003).

How Do People Obtain and Lose Health Insurance Coverage?

Most people choose to enroll in health insurance when it is offered on the job, including lower income workers and young adults who work. About two-thirds of Americans under age 65 are covered through employment-based plans offered at either their job or that of a parent or spouse (Fronstin, 2002).[5] Typically employees and their employer share the cost of coverage. Nearly seven percent of Americans under age 65, including some lower income people, purchase their own individual or family policies from the private, nongroup insurance market. About 15 percent are covered by public insurance (primarily Medicaid) (Fronstin, 2002). When parents are insured, whether they are in single- or two-parent families, more than 95 percent of the time all of their children are also covered (IOM, 2002b). Medicare covers nearly all individuals over age 65 (Mills and Bhandari, 2003).

Despite the variety of paths to coverage (employment, public programs, individual purchase), 17.2 percent of working-age Americans and children remain uninsured (Mills and Bhandari, 2003). Roughly one-fourth of workers have not been offered coverage by their employer, and half of these remain uninsured (Custer and Ketsche, 2000b). Some with a workplace offer report that they cannot afford the out-of-pocket or employee's share of the premium. Insurance is becoming increasingly expensive for employers of low-wage workers and those with small firms to offer the *benefit* and for workers to accept coverage when it is offered (Thorpe and Florence, 1999; Chernew et al., 2002; Kaiser/HRET, 2003). For a cohort of adults between ages 21 and 60 that was followed for four years (1996–2000), a job change or loss of a job was more often the reason for becoming uninsured than was the loss of public coverage. Those experiencing an uninsured spell were more likely than average to be young, African American or Latino,

---

[5]Some people report multiple sources of coverage, for example, they may have Medicaid for part of a year and a workplace policy at another time. Therefore, adding together employment-based, individual, and public insurance coverage rates yield more than the 83.5 percent of the U.S. population with some form of coverage during the year.

How People Gain Coverage

- Get a job where insurance is offered and premiums are affordable
- Purchase insurance on your own, if you qualify and can afford the premiums
- Marry someone with insurance and if family out-of-pocket premiums are affordable
- Qualify for Medicaid, SCHIP, or Medicare

How People Lose Coverage

- Lose a job where insurance was offered, so employer no longer subsidizes premiums
- Lose Medicaid or SCHIP eligibility once you or your children grow up or if your family's income increases
- Lose your spouse due to separation, divorce, or death
- Attain the age of 19 or graduate from college and lose eligibility under parents' plan
- Your insurer goes out of business or cancels its contract with you, or your employer denies coverage to you
- Be priced out of the market when the cost of premiums increases

FIGURE 2.1 Gaining and losing coverage.
SOURCE: IOM, 2001a.

lower waged, less well educated (high school graduate or less), and from a lower income household (Kuttner and McLaughlin, 2003). Federal reforms, such as the Health Insurance Portability and Accountability Act of 1996, have established limited rights to purchase individual plans for those formerly covered by employment-based insurance but do not regulate the size of the premium that might be charged (Nichols and Blumberg, 1998; IOM, 2001a).

People can lose coverage when they change jobs or become unemployed, when life circumstances shift, or when rising premiums make insurance unaffordable (IOM, 2001a); see Figure 2.1. When a worker with employment-based coverage reaches age 65, retires, and qualifies for Medicare, a younger spouse may be left without coverage. When children turn 19 years old, generally the age limit for coverage as a dependent, they must purchase a separate, individual health insurance policy unless they are still in school or become uninsured. While teenagers or those graduating from college may be ready to go to work, they are less likely than their older coworkers to find jobs that include health benefits or to earn enough to purchase insurance independently (Quinn et al., 2000; IOM, 2001a; Collins et al., 2003). Some young, healthy people may choose to take the risk rather than buy coverage. Marriage is associated with job and career choices that lead to an increased likelihood of having employment-based health insurance for the whole family. Becoming separated, divorced, or widowed are other examples of life transitions that can increase the risk that family members will lose their employment-based coverage.

What Are the Barriers to Insuring People Under the Current System?

Health insurance eligibility, enrollment in a plan, and maintenance of enrollment depend on many interdependent factors, including the local labor market and health services, state regulatory and program policies, demographics, consumer knowledge, and personal choices (see Figure 2.2). Health insurance may or may not be available to an employer depending on its size and type of industry; a firm may or may not offer a policy that its employees perceive to be affordable; an individual applying for a nongroup policy may or may not be healthy enough to qualify or be able to afford the risk-adjusted premium; and public programs may have more or less restrictive eligibility standards. Every state and locality has a particular configuration of characteristics, including its industrial base, regulatory environment, demographics, and public programs, that ultimately affects the opportunities for coverage and results in more or fewer people having health insurance.

Affordability of Premiums

As a group, those who lack health insurance most often share the perception that coverage is unaffordable. This is not to say, however, that health insurance becomes "affordable" across the board at a given premium cost or income level (Bundorf and Pauly, 2002; Levy and DeLeire, 2002). Although two-thirds of all people without coverage have incomes below 200 percent of FPL, some individuals and families with relatively low incomes do take up employer offers of coverage and some relatively high-income individuals and families forgo coverage (IOM, 2001a; Bundorf and Pauly, 2002). Nonetheless, unaffordability is the top reason uninsured adults give for why they are uninsured (Hoffman and Schlobohm, 2000), as well as the major reason employed persons turn down coverage when their employer offers it (Cooper and Schone, 1997; Thorpe and Florence, 1999; Cutler, 2002). Most uninsured families would not have sufficient funds in their budget to purchase health insurance without a substantial premium subsidy (IOM, 2001a, 2002a).

The high cost of premiums is also the most common reason small firms give for not offering health insurance (Kaiser/HRET, 2003). Small employers often receive poorer benefits for premiums comparable to larger firms. Administrative costs and expenses other than benefits are usually 10 percent of premiums for large employers but 20 to 25 percent for small employers (GAO, 2001).

Medical Underwriting and Denial of Coverage

Medical underwriting practices applied to individual applicants for nongroup coverage are necessarily sensitive to an applicant's health status, age, family income, and geographic area in order to protect the insurer from expected risks

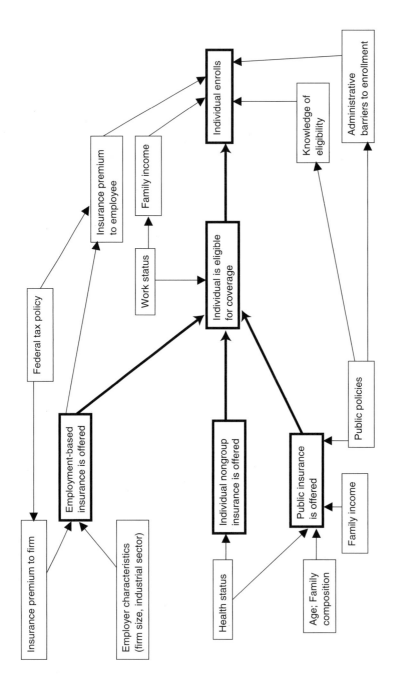

FIGURE 2.2 Factors affecting eligibility and enrollment.
NOTE: Bold lines indicate major pathways and decision points.
SOURCE: IOM, 2001a.

(Chollet and Kirk, 1998). Medical underwriting directly affects only those who purchase health insurance in the individual market. Nonetheless it is a significant barrier to coverage for some of the people most likely to benefit from coverage because of their relatively high expected use. Medical underwriting is inevitable in a competitive market with small and voluntary *risk pools*. Whereas young and healthy people face below-average premium prices, an older person or someone in poor health may face prohibitively high premiums. One study of eight nongroup insurance markets found that persons with health problems were quoted a premium price nearly 40 percent higher than were otherwise comparable potential buyers without health problems (Pollitz et al., 2001). In addition, most states allow risk rating by age, making individual policies relatively expensive for older people (Chollet and Kirk, 1998; Blue Cross Blue Shield Association, 2000). Still, because older people highly value having health insurance, they are more likely to purchase it in the *nongroup or individual market* than are younger adults. Some 29 states have established *high-risk pools* for persons who are uninsurable in the individual market because their poor health puts them at risk for incurring large health care bills. However, there are often waiting lists or closed enrollments as well as high premiums (GAO, 1996; Achman and Chollet, 2001).

Eligibility Restrictions for Public Programs

Public programs such as Medicaid and the State Children's Health Insurance Program (SCHIP) provide coverage for specific categories of the poor who tend to be excluded from the employment-based approach to financing health services delivery. The combination of strict eligibility requirements and complex enrollment procedures often makes public coverage difficult to obtain and even more difficult to maintain over time. Qualifying to participate in public programs involves fulfilling requirements related to income and assets (so-called means testing), being a member of a specific group that is eligible for benefits (e.g., pregnant women, minor children, or disabled), and meeting immigration status and residency requirements. Eligibility requirements vary from state to state.

Medicaid and SCHIP eligibility and enrollment policies are also subject to fluctuating fiscal conditions for the states that administer these programs, with more expansive eligibility and outreach to potential participants in better economic and fiscal times and cutbacks in eligibility and enrollment efforts during periods of fiscal stress (Howell et al., 2002; Smith and Ellis, 2002; Nathanson and Ku, 2003).

Is the Uninsured Population Growing?

Over the past 25 years, growth in the number of uninsured Americans has exceeded the rate of growth in the population under 65 years, despite an increasingly tight labor market that expanded employment-based coverage and yielded tax revenues to expand public coverage programs (IOM, 2001a). With the current combination of higher unemployment, rapidly rising costs of health care and insurance premiums, and state budget problems, absent major public policy reforms, the national uninsured rate will rise more rapidly in future years (Chernew et al., 2002; Cutler, 2002).

Looking forward, one study of the impact of different economic scenarios estimated that

• "Assuming continued economic growth and moderate health care cost inflation, the number of uninsured Americans will rise to more than 48 million in 2009.
• In the event of a recession, the number who lack coverage will reach 61 million by 2009.
• Rapid economic growth, coupled with rapid health care cost inflation such as characterized the 1980s, would lead to roughly 55 million uninsured in 2009" (Custer and Ketsche, 2000, p. 3).

Even without growth in the overall numbers, there is substantial variation in state and local uninsured rates, median durations of uninsured spells of individuals, and sizes and concentrations of uninsured groups within different populations (IOM, 2001a). This varied concentration of uninsured populations means that some adverse effects of uninsurance can be more severe in certain communities than would be expected from the national averaged data discussed in the section above.

ASSESSING THE EFFECTS OF HEALTH
INSURANCE ON HEALTH-RELATED OUTCOMES

Isolating and measuring the independent effect of having or lacking health insurance is an analytic challenge because virtually all studies are observational and many characteristics that vary with health insurance status, including income, education, race and ethnicity, and health behaviors, also affect individual health outcomes. Figure 2.3 outlines the mechanisms by which health insurance influences the amount and kind of health care received and a person's health outcomes. Coverage facilitates receipt of health care services that can improve personal health.

Uninsured people are less likely to have any medical contact and on average have fewer visits for care than people with either public or private coverage. Thus opportunities for detecting the presence of an illness or forestalling the progression of a chronic condition like diabetes are missed. Patients are also less likely to have a regular source of care to coordinate their health care or to have high-quality, evidence-based care. When the uninsured receive care in hospitals, their care management, even for trauma or premature birth, differs from that of insured patients, with uninsured patients receiving less intensive services (Hadley, 2002; IOM, 2002b).

This section summarizes the Committee's findings about the effect of health

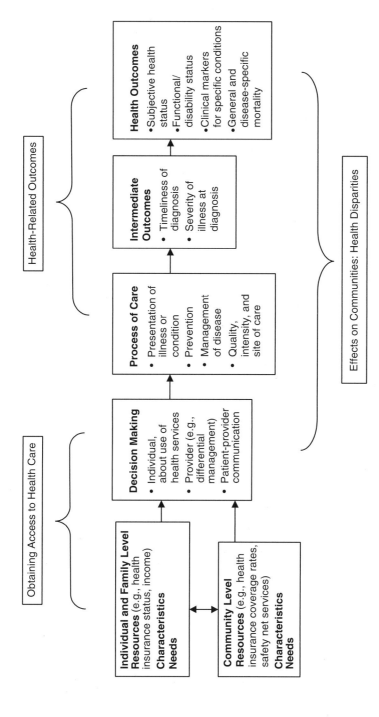

FIGURE 2.3 A conceptual framework for assessing the effect of health insurance status on health-related outcomes for adults.
SOURCE: IOM, 2002a.

insurance on a spectrum of health-related outcomes. These findings were drawn from methodologically sound research studies and natural experiments in which states extended health care coverage.[6]

Does Lack of Insurance Impede Access to and Use of Health Care?

Without coverage, the uninsured—whether children, pregnant women, or other adults—receive fewer services than their insured counterparts or no care at all (IOM, 2002a, b). They are less likely to have any physician visit within a year or establish a "medical home" with a regular source of primary care. They receive, on average, fewer preventive health services, less regular care for management of chronic diseases, and poorer care in the hospital.

Lesser Use and Lack of Preventive Health Services for Children and Adults

Uninsured children use medical and dental services less frequently and are less likely to get their prescriptions filled than insured children, even after taking into account differences in family income, race and ethnicity, and health status (Newacheck et al., 1998b; McCormick et al., 2001; IOM, 2002b). They are less likely to receive routine, preventive well-child checkups and immunizations. Half of uninsured children have not had a doctor's visit in the past year, more than twice the rate of privately insured children (McCormick et al., 2001).

Adolescents as a group are particularly at risk of not having any physician visits in the past year or a regular source of care. Their need for some kinds of health care services, such as mental health screening and treatment for drinking and other risky behaviors, increases in their late teenage years, yet 17 percent of adolescents ages 15 to 17 are uninsured, the highest rate of all children (McCormick et al., 2001). Over one-quarter (27.4 percent) of adolescents ages 10 to 18 in families earning less than the federal poverty standard are uninsured (Newacheck et al., 1999). Forty-four percent of young adults aged 19-29 are uninsured at least part of the year. Though generally a healthy population, young adults are particularly vulnerable to injuries, HIV, and pregnancy, but when uninsured their regular access to the health system is disrupted (Collins et al., 2003).

Uninsured women receive fewer prenatal care services than their insured counterparts and report greater difficulty in obtaining the care they believe they

---

[6]The Committee based its findings and conclusions on studies that adjusted for basic social, demographic, and health characteristics. In health outcomes studies, unless otherwise noted, health insurance status was measured at baseline and does not reflect duration of coverage or period of uninsurance. Appendix B in *Care Without Coverage* and Appendix C in *Health Insurance Is a Family Matter* summarize the studies reviewed by the Committee.

need. In 1996 and 1997, 15 percent of uninsured pregnant women had no prenatal visit compared with 4 percent of women with private or public coverage (Bernstein, 1999). Other studies find large differences in use between privately insured and uninsured women and smaller differences between uninsured and publicly insured women (IOM, 2002b). Uninsured women in labor are less likely to receive clinically indicated cesarean section deliveries for risks like breech presentation, fetal distress, or failure of labor to progress than are similar women who have coverage (Aron et al., 2000). Uninsured adults are also less likely to receive preventive health services such as mammograms, clinical breast exams, Pap tests, and colorectal screening (Powell-Griner et al., 1999; Ayanian et al., 2000; Breen et al., 2001).

Less Access to a Regular Source of Care

Maintaining an ongoing relationship with a specific provider who keeps records, manages care, and is available for consultation between visits is a key to high-quality care (O'Connor et al., 1998; IOM, 2001b). When children or adults have health insurance, they are more likely to have a regular provider who watches out for their health. People with insurance are more likely to see the same doctor at their usual source of care, and insurance status is the most important factor in white-Hispanic health differences in access to care (Hargraves and Hadley, 2003). The likelihood that someone who is uninsured lacks a regular source of care has increased substantially over the past several decades (Zuvekas and Weinick, 1999; Weinick et al., 2000). Even if people have health insurance that does not cover preventive services, they are more likely to receive appropriate services than are those without any form of health insurance, partly because they are more likely to have a regular source of care (IOM, 2002a).

Uninsured children are more likely to obtain routine and sick care from different sources, such as hospital clinics and health centers, than insured children, who are more likely to be treated in the physician's office (Holl et al., 1995). Well-child care and a regular care provider are important for monitoring children's development and detecting potential problems early before they can cause long-term health consequences. Children without insurance were more than three times as likely as children with Medicaid coverage to have no regular source of care (15 percent versus 5 percent), and uninsured adults were more than three times as likely as either privately or publicly insured adults to lack a regular source of care (35 percent versus 11 percent) (Haley and Zuckerman, 2000).

Uninsured children with special health needs are particularly disadvantaged because they require considerably more than routine care. One out of every nine children with special needs (roughly the same rate as among all children) remains uninsured (Newacheck et al., 1998a). Uninsured children with special health needs are less likely to have a usual source of care, less likely to have seen a doctor in the previous year, and less likely to get needed medical, mental health, dental or vision care, or prescriptions than are those with insurance.

Identifying chronic conditions early and providing evidence-based, cost-effective interventions on an ongoing and coordinated basis can improve health outcomes. Yet uninsured adults with chronic conditions are less likely to have a usual source of care than a chronically ill person with coverage (Ayanian et al., 2000; Fish-Parcham, 2001). Nineteen percent of uninsured adults with heart disease and 13 percent with hypertension lack a usual source of care, compared with 8 and 4 percent respectively of their insured counterparts (Fish-Parcham, 2001).

Differential Management in Hospital-Based Care

Uninsured patients who are hospitalized for any of a number of conditions are more likely to receive fewer services and, when admitted, are more likely to experience substandard care and resultant injury than are insured patients (Burstin et al., 1992). Some of the differences in care and outcomes between insured and uninsured hospital patients may stem from differences in the site of care. For example, a study of maternity patients in San Francisco revealed that privately insured women at a high risk of complications were much more likely to deliver at a hospital with neonatal intensive care facilities than were uninsured women (Phibbs et al., 1993). One statewide study found that uninsured sick newborns average shorter hospital stays and receive fewer inpatient services even after controlling for race, ethnicity, diagnoses, and hospital characteristics (Braveman et al., 1991).

Uninsured adults can experience treatment differences as well. For example, uninsured women with breast cancer are less likely than privately insured women to receive breast-conserving surgery even when stage of diagnosis is taken into account (Roetzheim et al., 2000a). Uninsured patients with acute myocardial infarction who met expert panel criteria for revascularization were less likely to be transferred to a hospital that performed this procedure: 91 percent of Medicare patients, 82 percent of privately insured patients, 75 percent of Medicaid patients, and just 53 percent of uninsured patients received this indicated surgery (Leape et al., 1999).

Does Lack of Insurance Impede Access to High-Quality, Evidence-Based Care?

The difference health insurance makes is not just in increasing utilization but also in ensuring appropriate care. Although not all of the care that insured populations use is necessary and appropriate (IOM, 2001b), overall, the care received by those with coverage contributes to health outcomes better than those experienced by otherwise comparable uninsured populations who on average receive many fewer and less appropriate services. People without health insurance are at a disadvantage in obtaining high-quality, evidence-based care recommended by professional groups. When appropriate care is not obtained, patients' health is placed at risk, conditions can become more severe, and the effects can linger. Increased severity frequently demands more intense treatment (e.g., hospitalization).

Less Likely to Receive Professionally Recommended Standard of Care

Uninsured adults are less likely than those with health insurance to receive preventive and screening services at the frequencies recommended by the U.S. Preventive Services Task Force (Powell-Griner et al., 1999; Ayanian et al., 2000; Breen et al., 2001). Even after adjustments for age, race, education, and regular source of care, uninsured adults are less likely to receive timely screening for breast, cervical, or colorectal cancer. The positive effect of having insurance is more evident with relatively costly preventive services such as mammograms than with less expensive ones such as Pap smears, for example (Zambrana et al., 1999; Cummings et al., 2000).

Uninsured adults living with chronic diseases are less likely to receive care for chronic health conditions that meets professionally recommended standards than are those who have health insurance. For example, uninsured adults with diabetes are less likely to receive regular foot or dilated eye exams that are important in the prevention of foot ulcers and blindness (Beckles et al., 1998). Uninsured patients with end-stage renal disease began dialysis at a later stage of their disease and with poorer clinical measures (e.g., more likely to be anemic) (Kausz et al., 2000).

Persons diagnosed with a mental illness who lack health insurance are less likely to receive mental health services than are those with any health insurance (Cooper-Patrick et al., 1999; McAlpine and Mechanic, 2000). Furthermore, having health insurance that covers mental health services increases the likelihood that the care received will be in accordance with professional practice guidelines (Wang et al., 2000).

Less Likely to Receive Medications That Are the Standard of Treatment

Lack of insurance can interfere with access to appropriate medications for controlling medical conditions. For example, uninsured adults with HIV infection were less likely to receive the highly effective medications shown to improve survival and that have become the standard of treatment (Carpenter et al., 1996, 1998; Goldman et al., 2001). Uninsured adults had less frequent monitoring of blood pressure once they were diagnosed with hypertension and were less likely to stay on recommended drug therapy than insured adults with hypertension (Huttin et al., 2000; Fish-Parcham, 2001).

Receiving Care in Less Appropriate Settings

The lack of timely screening services and preventive care leads to poor health outcomes because of delayed diagnoses and failure to control treatable conditions. When they finally receive treatment, those without health insurance are more likely to require more expensive services because of deteriorating health. For example, uninsured patients are more likely to develop severe uncontrolled hypertension requiring emergency admission to the hospital than are insured patients (Shea et al., 1992a, b).

Other conditions (e.g., asthma; ear, nose, and throat infections; pneumonia; diabetes) also are best treated early; without timely outpatient care, unnecessary hospitalizations occur. Expansion of SCHIP in Pennsylvania has shown that as the portion of children receiving physician visits increased, emergency room visits decreased (Lave et al., 1998). Expansion of Medicaid coverage also has been shown to reduce potentially avoidable hospitalizations among children (Dafny and Gruber, 2000).

What Are the Health Consequences for Individuals and Their Families?

Ascertaining whether health insurance improves health outcomes is critical to shaping public policy about health insurance and the financing of health care more generally. Uninsured people are more likely to receive too little medical care and to receive it too late, to be sicker, and to die sooner.

Direct measures of health outcomes include self-reported health status, mortality, stage of disease at time of diagnosis, and physiologic measures (e.g., controlled blood pressure in persons with hypertension). Research studies consistently show that working-age Americans (those between 18 and 65) who do not have health insurance have poorer health and die prematurely. For children, their health is diminished and their long-term development is at risk when they are not covered.

Diminished Health-Related Quality of Life

Adults in late middle age are more likely to experience declines in function and health status if they lack or lose health insurance coverage (Baker et al., 2001). Changes in health status might include worsening control of blood pressure, decreased ability to walk or climb stairs, or decline of general self-perceived wellness and functioning. The effect of being uninsured on self-reported health measures is greater for lower income persons (Franks et al., 1993b). Another example is the deterioration in *health-related quality of life* reported for uninsured men with prostate cancer during treatment. They are more likely to have a delayed diagnosis, unlike men with either public or private insurance (Roetzheim et al., 1999; Penson et al., 2001).

Developmental Risks for Children

For children, using health care services routinely and appropriately is considered a positive health outcome in its own right because well-child care has been demonstrated to be effective in enhancing longer term health and development.

Health conditions that are readily treatable and that could affect a child's long-term development and life chances if untreated are more likely to go undetected when children are not insured. Conditions such as asthma, iron deficiency anemia, and middle-ear infections, if left untreated or improperly controlled, can affect mental development and school performance, language development, and hearing (IOM, 2002b). For example, there is an increased likelihood of mild or moderate mental retardation associated with iron deficiency anemia; approximately 9 percent of toddlers, 9 to 11 percent of adolescent girls, and 11 percent of women of childbearing age are iron deficient (Looker et al., 1997). Although long-term studies linking insurance status to these conditions and later life outcomes have not been conducted, uninsured children are at greater risk of such undetected conditions because of their lack of routine care.

Increased Risk for Adverse Events

For the five disease conditions that the Committee studied (diabetes, cardiovascular disease, end-stage renal disease, HIV infection, and mental illness), uninsured adults have consistently worse clinical outcomes than do insured patients. For example, uncontrolled blood glucose levels, which put diabetics at increased risk of hospitalization and additional complications (e.g., heart and kidney disease) and disability (e.g., amputations and blindness), are more frequent for uninsured adults (IOM, 2002a).

In addition, uninsured pregnant women are more likely to have adverse maternal outcomes, such as pregnancy-related hypertension and placental abruption, than privately insured women. Improved maternal outcomes, however, may require enhanced services such as counseling and other enabling services in addition to health insurance (Weis, 1992; Haas et al., 1993; IOM, 2002b).

Decreased Life Expectancy for Newborns and Children

Uninsured newborns are more likely than insured newborns to have poorer health outcomes such as low birthweight, which is a risk factor for developmental problems. Uninsured babies are also more likely to die prematurely. Measures across entire geographic populations, however, yield mixed evidence of improvement in health outcomes as a result of increased health insurance rates (IOM, 2002b). State experiments in Washington and California have found better birth outcomes in terms of birthweight and prematurity when additional services such as targeted case management, psychosocial and nutritional counseling, and other services were made available (Homan and Korenbrot, 1998; Salganicoff and Wyn, 1999). Insurance coverage as a result of Medicaid eligibility extensions in the 1980s and 1990s was associated with reductions in child mortality after the first year of life (Currie and Gruber, 1996a). At the same time, insurance coverage without enhanced prenatal services has not always yielded improvements in neonatal outcomes (Baldwin et al., 1998; Marquis and Long, 2002).

Pediatric trauma patients with private insurance have less risk of in-hospital mortality than the uninsured, even after adjusting for injury severity (Li and Davis, 2001). Uninsured children are estimated to be 40 percent less likely to receive medical attention for serious injuries than insured children, regardless of their race or ethnicity (Overpeck et al., 1997).

Decreased Life Expectancy Among Adults

The Committee has estimated that uninsured adults have age-specific mortality rates approximately 25 percent higher than those of privately insured adults, based upon its extensive review of health outcomes studies and as estimated in longitudinal studies of overall mortality that adjust for multiple sociodemographic and health-related characteristics (Franks et al., 1993a; Sorlie et al., 1994; Hadley, 2002; IOM, 2002a). The Committee estimated that, for the year 2000, an estimated 18,000 excess deaths among adults between ages 25 and 64 could be attributed to lack of coverage (IOM, 2002a). The 18,000 excess deaths annually associated with uninsurance are comparable in magnitude to the 17,500 estimated deaths from diabetes and 19,000 deaths from cerebrovascular disease (stroke) in 2001 among the population under age 65. Also, there were 14,100 HIV deaths and 19,700 homicides among the total population that year.

Uninsured people who have cancer, HIV, or cardiovascular disease or who are victims of car crashes have worse mortality experience than do insured people with these conditions. Uninsured cancer patients are more likely to die prematurely than persons with insurance largely because of delayed diagnosis. This evidence comes from population-based research using area or statewide cancer registries for breast, cervical, colorectal, and prostate cancer and melanoma (IOM, 2002a). For example, uninsured women with breast cancer have a risk of dying that is between 30 and 50 percent higher than the risk for women with private health insurance (Ayanian et al., 1993; Lee-Feldstein et al., 2000; Roetzheim et al., 2000a), and uninsured patients with colorectal cancer are about 50 percent more likely to die than are patients with private coverage, even when the cancer is diagnosed at similar stages (Roetzheim et al., 2000b).

Uninsured adults are at greater risk of premature death, reflecting the fact that they receive fewer screening services for serious illnesses such as cancer and less intensive and effective treatment for acute conditions such as traumatic injury and heart attacks. In one statewide study of hospitalized car crash victims, uninsured patients were found to receive less care and had a 37 percent higher mortality rate than did privately insured patients (Doyle, 2001). Having health insurance of any kind has been found to reduce mortality in HIV-infected adults by 71 to 85 percent over a 6-month period, with the greater reduction found for a more recent time period during which effective drug therapies were in more widespread use (Goldman et al., 2001). Uninsured patients with acute cardiovascular disease are less likely to be admitted to a hospital that performs angiography or revascularization procedures, are less likely to receive these diagnostic and treatment procedures, and are more likely to die in the short term (IOM, 2002a). Health insurance reduces the disparity in receipt of these services for women relative to men and for members of racial and ethnic minority groups (Carlisle et al., 1997; Daumit et al., 1999, 2000).

What Are the Health Effects of Discontinuous Coverage?

Health insurance is most likely to improve health outcomes if coverage is continuous rather than intermittent and if it links people to appropriate health care. Adults with intermittent or no health insurance coverage experience greater declines in health status over time than do adults with continuous coverage. Being uninsured for relatively short periods (1 to 4 years) appears to result in a decrease in general health status (Lurie et al., 1984, 1986; Baker et al., 2001).

If Americans were to become insured on a continuous basis, their health would be expected to improve. The survival benefits derived from insurance coverage, however, can be achieved in full only when health insurance is acquired well before the development of advanced disease. The problem of later diagnosis and higher mortality among uninsured women with breast cancer, for example, cannot be solved by insuring women once their disease is diagnosed (Perkins et al., 2001).

Discontinuity affects access to health care and outcomes. For example, 25 percent of adults with diabetes went without a checkup within the past two years when they were uninsured for a year or more, compared to 7 percent of diabetics who were uninsured for less than a year and 5 percent of diabetics with health insurance (Beckles et al., 1998; Ayanian et al., 2000). Lacking health insurance for longer periods increases the risk of uncontrolled blood sugar levels in persons with diabetes, which, over time, put them at risk for additional chronic disease and disability. Similarly, discontinuity of insurance disrupts therapeutic relationships for persons with hypertension and worsens blood pressure control (Carlisle et al., 1997; Daumit et al., 1999, 2000).

Children with gaps in health insurance coverage have less access to health services than do those with continuous coverage. For example, after expansion of SCHIP in New York, immunization rates rose, with the greatest increase among previously uninsured children and those who had a gap in coverage longer than six months (Rodewald et al., 1997). The improved immunization rate followed the shift in provision of immunizations from public health departments to health care providers whose coordination of care for the children served as a medical home for their patients.

Generally, patients with private insurance have the best outcomes, while the uninsured have the highest proportion of late-stage diagnoses, with intermediate outcomes for Medicaid enrollees. However, some studies find that Medicaid enrollees' outcomes are more comparable to the uninsured. The latter may stem in part from the frequent transitions to uninsured status that many Medicaid enrollees experience and the resulting interruptions likely to occur in the use of health services (Perkins et al., 2001; IOM, 2002a). Coverage is particularly episodic for lower income women. Medicaid enrollment periods for single women tend to be short and may depend on pregnancy status. More than half maintain enrollment for less than a year, not quite one-third last more than two years, and just 15 percent remain enrolled for five years (Short and Freedman, 1998). These medical consequences of coverage gaps will be discussed in the context of the structure of health insurance later in this chapter.

FAMILY AND COMMUNITY EFFECTS OF UNINSURANCE

Health insurance serves multiple constituencies and distinct purposes. For individuals and families, insurance is one means to promote health and plan for, if not prevent, exceptional health care costs. Providers of health care benefit from insurance as a reliable source of payment. Employers offer health benefits to attract workers and retain a satisfied and productive workforce. Communities benefit from a healthier population and potentially more stable health care institutions.

Uninsurance can have effects that extend beyond uninsured persons and their families to community health care institutions, providers, and even the insured population. For example, a hospital outpatient department that serves an increasing number of uninsured patients without commensurate increases in financial support for uncompensated care may discontinue costly services, affecting access for everyone in the community. Although study of community-level effects of uninsurance is relatively recent, and the Committee has outlined additional needed research in this area, the evidence that is available justifies the immediate adoption of policies to address the lack of health insurance (IOM, 2003a).

What Are the Financial Repercussions of Uninsurance for Families?

Families with at least one uninsured member are predominantly lower income families. To be able to pay for rent, food, and other necessities, poor families have to decide between paying insurance premiums or forgoing coverage and paying out of pocket for health care services when necessary (Levy and DeLiere, 2002). Figure 2.4 shows how the cost of a full premium for an average employment-based benefit for family coverage compares with family income.

High Out-of-Pocket Expenses Despite Doing Without Care

Because of concerns about the associated costs, uninsured families are parsimonious in their use of health services. On average, families with some or all members uninsured are more likely to report using *no* health services. Those that use some services use fewer than do families with all members covered by private insurance (IOM, 2002b). Thus, it is not surprising that they spend on average less

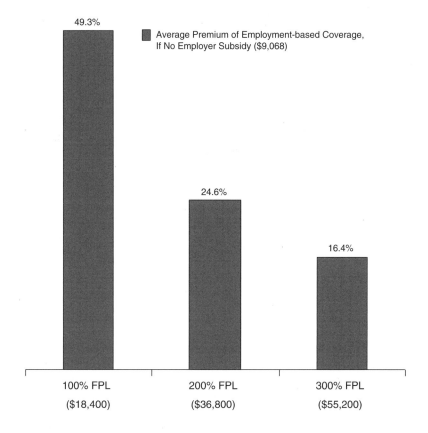

FIGURE 2.4 Share of a four-person family's income compared to premium costs to purchase family coverage in 2003.
SOURCES: Kaiser/HRET, 2003; DHHS, 2003.

on health care in absolute dollars. However, out-of-pocket health expenditures are a higher portion of family income than they are in insured families. In families with some members covered, out-of-pocket expenses relative to income still exceed that of fully insured families.

Even in the healthiest of families, if one member has an accident or a costly hospital stay, the resulting medical bills can affect the economic stability of the whole family. Uninsured patients are likely to be charged more than those with insurance because they do not have a large insurer to negotiate a discount (Miller, 2003). The cost to a patient of hospital admission in 1999 for simple pneumonia in an adult might be $100 to $3,434 for a *fee-for-service* plan, but $9,812 for a person with no insurance (IOM, 2001a). As the time without health insurance lengthens, families continue to gamble with their financial security as well as their health.

Even brief periods without coverage expose families to the financial risk of incurring extraordinarily high medical expenses for an incident like a car crash or treatment for cancer.

Potential for Bankruptcy

How do families cope with the burden of medical bills? Some families delay payment and may be dunned by collections agents. Families with uninsured members have fewer assets than do fully insured families and are less likely to have the capacity to borrow to cover major unexpected health care costs. More than half of all working-age adults uninsured currently or in the recent past reported difficulties paying medical bills, compared with less than a quarter of insured adults (Duchon et al., 2001). Of those with severe bill problems, two-thirds reported borrowing from family or a friend and a quarter needed a loan or mortgage on their home in order to pay (Duchon et al., 2001). Some families resort to declaring bankruptcy and put their future credit rating in jeopardy. Medical bills are a factor in nearly half of all bankruptcy filings, but it is not known whether bankruptcy is more likely for uninsured families than for those with coverage (Jacoby et al., 2000).

Who Pays for the Care of Uninsured Persons?

When a family is uninsured and cannot pay all its medical bills, the financial burden falls on the providers of services and on the broader community, through a variety of public and private mechanisms. Persons who are uninsured for the full year pay 35 percent, on average, of the overall cost of medical services they receive (Hadley and Holahan, 2003a; IOM, 2003a). The amount paid out of pocket varies by type of service. For example, uninsured individuals pay for nearly all (88 percent) of their prescription medications but for only 7 percent on average of hospital expenses they incur (AHRQ, 2001). Supports for care to uninsured patients come from federal, state, and local programs and grants; from organized philanthropy; and from the donated services and uncompensated care absorbed by providers.

There is no uniform public responsibility to subsidize or pay for the care delivered to uninsured persons. The public sector financed between 75 and 85 percent of $35 billion in *uncompensated care* estimated to have been rendered to uninsured persons in 2001 (Hadley and Holahan, 2003a). The size of the lower income population (families with incomes less than 200 percent of FPL) in an area determines the relative need for public support for health care of all kinds (including both insurance and direct services) (Holahan and Pohl, 2003). The financing that exists is spread unevenly and varies by locality, not necessarily matching local needs for care (IOM, 2003a). The financial and organizational relationships between safety net arrangements and mainstream health care imply that unreimbursed expenditures for health services delivered to uninsured persons are borne by both public and private payers and by federal taxpayers as well as state and local ones.

Private payers (e.g., employers, insurers) and private-sector health care providers (e.g., nonprofit hospitals, physician practices) are widely assumed to *cross-subsidize* the costs of care for uninsured patients. Over the past 25 years, public policies to control health care costs and increasingly competitive health care markets have constrained payment rates. As a result, opportunities for private cross-subsidy of uncompensated care have eroded. The existence of such subsidies is difficult to document. Most analysts believe the opportunities for such *cost shifting* declined during the past decade (IOM, 2003a). Over the same period, the proportion of physicians who provided *charity care* (whether to uninsured or insured persons) declined, a decrease that is explained as a response to reduced provider revenues (Reed et al., 2001; Cunningham et al., 1999).

Does the Size of the Uninsured Population Matter for Access to Care in a Community?

The effects of uninsurance on communities have been felt most strongly in communities with large or growing uninsured populations, particularly in central urban neighborhoods and in rural areas, and in parts of the health care system such as public hospitals that serve many uninsured persons (IOM, 2003a). Programs to provide and pay for uninsured care are often stretched to their resource limits, with existing dollars outstripped by the perceived health needs of the population (Lewin and Altman, 2000; Felt-Lisk et al., 2001; IOM, 2003a). Health care providers who treat a large number of uninsured patients are likely to accumulate uncompensated costs that may impair their ability to continue delivering care. The Committee's exploratory analyses of uninsurance effects on the availability of hospital services and hospital financial margins could not capture and do not reflect differences in the strategic behavior of hospitals in response to uninsured populations, differences that affect the relative shares of uninsured patients at different facilities in the same community. Not all hospitals, even those in communities with high uninsurance rates, serve a high or growing number of uninsured patients, and hospitals that do serve large numbers have varied experiences, depending on corporate resources and the public supports and subsidies available to them (Gaskin, 1999; Catholic Hospital Association, 2002).

A high uninsured rate in a community can result in reduced access to clinic-based primary care, specialty health services, and hospital-based care, particularly emergency medical services and trauma care (IOM, 2003a). It may also result in reduced availability of other primary and preventive care services and the loss of community health care providers, including the closure of hospitals. Access to health services and consequent benefits may be compromised for others within the community beyond those who lack coverage. Even for healthy community members, having more advanced medical services and resources available has real value.

Reduced Availability of Clinic-Based Primary Care Services

Serving a high or increasing number of uninsured persons reduces a community health center's capacity to provide ambulatory care to all of its clients, insured as well as uninsured. The growing number of uninsured patients in community health centers, public health clinics, and other safety-net facilities may be due to referrals from other providers trying to reduce their uncompensated care burden (Hawkins and Rosenbaum, 1998). Community clinics face financial pressures with reduced income from Medicaid patients (especially due to managed care contracting), reduced public subsidies, and an increased portion of their population that is uninsured (Lewin and Altman, 2000). The loss of ambulatory care clinic services is particularly damaging to vulnerable populations because these clinics serve a higher proportion of low-income and minority group members under age 65 and have safety-net missions (e.g., serving farmworkers, homeless persons) and patients with specific high-risk diagnoses (e.g., tuberculosis, substance abuse). A longitudinal study of 588 community health centers between 1996 and 1999 found that reductions in the scope of services and capacity to provide primary care were concentrated among health centers with a sizable uninsured population or a recent rapid increase in the number of uninsured clients that lessened the centers' ability to provide primary care (McAlearney, 2002).

Reduced Availability of Hospital-Based Care

Many hospitals operate with financial constraints that leave little room for cross-subsidizing the costs of uninsured patients. In urban areas the adverse financial effects on hospitals are more likely to have an impact on low-income residents (insured and uninsured) who have few options for care other than their local public or private safety-net hospitals. Inner city hospitals face pressure to cut their costs by cutting services. As a result, hospitals in urban areas with high uninsured rates have less total inpatient capacity, offer fewer services for vulnerable populations (such as AIDS care), and are less likely to offer trauma and burn care (Gaskin and Needleman, 2003; IOM, 2003a). Hospitals in neighboring areas without so many uninsured may continue to operate as usual (Draper et al., 2001a). In rural areas, there is less opportunity to segment the market, and the adverse effects of high uninsured rates on hospital operating margins are likely to affect the availability of services for all community residents (Sutton et al., 2001). Hospitals in rural areas with higher uninsured rates have fewer intensive care unit beds, offer fewer psychiatric inpatient services, and are less likely to offer high-technology services such as radiation therapy (IOM, 2003a; Needleman and Gaskin, 2003).

Emergency departments (EDs) and trauma centers are key examples of how market pressures and public policies interact in ways that create incentives for hospitals to reduce their exposure to financial losses associated with an "open door" policy to serve all comers without regard to their ability to pay. Rising use rates by the uninsured can worsen ED overcrowding and the financial status of ED operations. A recent survey of 1,501 hospitals finds that 62 percent report their EDs to be at or over capacity, often due to the inability to move seriously ill or injured patients into inpatient beds (Lewin Group, 2002). A survey of urban hospitals by the General Accounting Office finds that many are ill equipped to handle a large number of patients, such as the number who would be seen with a bioterrorism incident (GAO, 2003). By limiting the number of inpatient beds available, hospital administrators are better able to control admissions. When a backup is severe, patients may be diverted to other facilities. In the mean time, the ED is unavailable to the insured and uninsured alike. Members of medically underserved groups are particularly likely to suffer reduced access because they have fewer options to obtain primary care outside EDs (Felt-Lisk et al., 2001; Weinick et al., 2002).

Financial stresses for hospitals have also increased the difficulty of recruiting medical specialists to serve on on-call panels for emergency rooms as required under the federal Emergency Medical Treatment and Labor Act (EMTALA). For example, in Phoenix, AZ, which had a 17 percent uninsured rate in 2001, specialty physicians such as orthopedists and neurosurgeons ended their affiliations with emergency departments because of the expected lack of compensation due to the high number of uninsured patients (Draper et al., 2001b).

Similarly, a high proportion of uninsured patients places significant financial stress on regional trauma centers. Trauma center patients are already more likely to be uninsured than all hospital patients (Eastman et al., 1991). Hospitals may decline to open a trauma center or may decide to close one in response to this financial stress. The closure of a regional trauma center puts the health of everyone in a community at risk, whether insured or uninsured.

Difficulty Obtaining Referrals for Specialty Health Services

Relatively high uninsured rates are also associated with the decreased ability of primary care providers to obtain specialty referrals for patients who are members of medically underserved groups. For example, insured and uninsured rural residents already experience reduced access to specialty care. Increasing numbers of uninsured patients prompt more providers to leave the community because their practices are not financially viable (Ormond et al., 2000). A study of primary care providers in 20 community health centers in 10 states revealed difficulties for practitioners in high uninsured-rate areas in obtaining specialty referrals for all of their patients, not just the uninsured (Fairbrother et al., 2002). Urban safety-net hospitals and academic health centers also have been affected by increased numbers of uninsured patients. Under financial pressure, some facilities have cut out specialty services with poor rates of reimbursement, such as burn units, pediatric and neonatal intensive care units, and HIV/AIDS care (Gaskin, 1999; Commonwealth Fund, 2001).

Does the Size of the Uninsured Population Affect a Community's Economic and Fiscal Health?

Although it is clear that the economic vitality of a community affects insurance coverage rates, the Committee also hypothesizes the converse—that health insurance coverage rates can affect the economic fortunes of a community, primarily through financial impacts on health services providers and institutions (IOM, 2003a). A high uninsured rate likely reflects fewer employers offering coverage and a lower wage labor force. The tenuous financial viability of local health providers due to uninsurance additionally affects both service delivery and jobs. Each of these puts financial stress on communities that try to maintain services through higher local prices for health care services and higher local taxes. Alternately, cutting local support can result in more uninsured in the area and reduced service availability for all community residents.

During economic downturns, when growth in uninsured populations increases the demand for uncompensated care, state and local reductions in health care spending may reduce the flow of federal dollars (such as Medicaid matching funds) into a community. Local community institutions and programs tend to serve as providers of last resort.

The dispersion and concentration of uninsured populations across regions, states, counties, and cities and across urban, suburban, and rural areas vary widely (IOM, 2003a, Appendix B). While the national average uninsured rate for Americans under 65 years is 17.2 percent, the rates for the states range from 8.8 percent in Minnesota to a high of 28.4 percent in Texas (Mills and Bhandari, 2003). Within a single state there can be considerable variation. Among the 67 counties in Florida, the uninsured rate varies from 12 percent to 30 percent uninsured, with many counties significantly different from the state's overall rate of 16.8 percent (Lazarus et al., 2000).[7] This variable concentration implies that the adverse effects of uninsurance will be more or less severe locally than national or even state-level uninsured rates would suggest.

Compared with the tax burden of federally or federal-and-state financed health insurance (Medicare or Medicaid and SCHIP), the costs of uncompensated care for those without coverage fall more heavily on local health care providers and taxpayers (IOM, 2003a). Communities that are disproportionately affected by uninsurance, for example, those with a preponderance of lower-wage and service-sector jobs, likewise have a smaller tax base with which to address the health care needs of uninsured residents. State-level efforts can make a significant difference in

---

[7]The estimates of uninsurance for Florida and its counties were devised using methods and sample sizes different from the Census Bureau's Current Population Survey, which is the basis for the discussion of the range of uninsured rates among the states. Because of these differences, the estimates given for Florida, and for Colorado and Minnesota in the example that follows, are not comparable to CPS estimates. See Appendix B in *A Shared Destiny* for more details (IOM, 2003a).

the rate of uninsurance. In two states with comparable portions of residents lacking employment-based coverage (22 percent for Colorado and 18 percent for Minnesota), the state of Minnesota enrolled 45 percent of persons without employment-based coverage in public insurance compared to Colorado, which enrolled 19 percent. As a result, the uninsured rate is 10 percent in Minnesota, compared with 17 percent in Colorado (Holahan, 2002).

Does the Size of the Uninsured Population Affect the Physical Health of a Community?

The sheer number of uninsured persons in an area adds to the community burden of disease and disability because uninsured persons are more likely than their privately insured counterparts to have poorer health, to be at greater risk for some communicable diseases, and to draw on public health resources (IOM, 2003a).

Worse Health Status and More Preventable Hospitalizations

Geographic differences in self-reported health status among the states correlate with state uninsured rates (Holahan, 2002). For urban, suburban, and nonmetropolitan communities across the country, uninsured rates also correlate with the health status reported by residents. Community uninsurance rates converge with a number of other factors that affect access to care and health status, such as the proportion of the population that is lower income and the proportion that consists of racial and ethnic minorities (Shi, 2000, 2001; IOM, 2001a, 2002a). Although these geographic disparities in health status are certainly not entirely attributable to the lack of coverage, the uncompensated care demands on health care providers and population health impacts are greater in communities with high uninsured rates (IOM, 2003a).

Potentially avoidable hospitalizations (sometimes called ambulatory-care-sensitive conditions) serve as an indicator of adequate access to primary and regular care. Uninsured patients are more likely to experience avoidable hospitalizations than are privately insured patients when measured as the proportion of all hospitalizations (Pappas et al., 1997). Hospitalization rates for potentially avoidable hospitalizations are higher in communities that include greater proportions of lower income and uninsured residents, indicating both access problems and greater severity of illness (IOM, 2003a).

Increased Risk for Communicable Diseases

Areas with relatively high uninsured rates are likely to have a greater burden of vaccine-preventable and communicable diseases and disability. For example, underimmunization increases the vulnerability of entire communities to outbreaks of diseases such as measles, pertussis (whooping cough), flu, pneumonia, and other diseases (IOM, 2000). Childhood and adult immunization levels are positively correlated with having either public or private health insurance. When uninsured children received coverage under SCHIP in New York state, statewide immunization rates for young children increased (Rodewald et al., 1997).

Increased Burden on Public Health Resources

Competing demands on state and local health departments as providers of last resort and as guardians of public health can adversely affect their ability to perform both functions adequately (GAO, 2003; IOM, 2003a,c). Public health functions include disease and immunization surveillance, community-based health education and behavioral interventions, emergency preparedness, and environmental health. The need for population-based public health services is expected to be greater now; at the same time there are growing demands on health departments to provide or pay for safety-net services for the uninsured. A recent survey finds that more than one-quarter of local health departments serve as the only safety-net provider in their community (Keane et al., 2001). Budgets for population-based public health activities that benefit all members of the community frequently are squeezed by these demands.

CURRENT COSTS AND SOCIETAL COSTS ATTRIBUTABLE TO UNINSURANCE

As a society, we directly invest in the health of those who have health insurance through tax subsidies for private insurance and publicly sponsored coverage. We also spend substantial public resources for direct health care services for those who lack coverage, yet the uninsured continue to have worse health outcomes. By estimating the health services costs now incurred by the tens of millions of uninsured Americans and some of the incremental costs and benefits across society of extending coverage, we provide an economic baseline against which health insurance reform strategies can be measured.

What Are the Health Services Costs Now Borne by the Uninsured Themselves?

As described earlier in the chapter, the uninsured use fewer health services yet have higher average out-of-pocket health expenses as a proportion of family income when they do use services. When uninsured people use health care services, they are often charged substantially more than are insured patients, whose insurance company has negotiated discounts (Lagnado, 2003). Among families with no members insured during the entire year and incomes below the poverty level, more than one in four had out-of-pocket expenses that exceeded 5 percent of income in 1996 (Taylor et al., 2001b). Families with no insurance for any of its members for the full year were nearly twice as likely to exceed the 5 percent

TABLE 2.1 Out-of-Pocket Expenses as Percentage of Family Income, by Insurance Coverage and Duration, Non-Medicare Families, 1996[a]

	Families Exceeding Threshold (percent)	
	5% or More of Income	10% or More of Income
All members insured for entire year	8.8	3.0
Some members uninsured and/or some period without health insurance	10.7	4.6
All members uninsured for entire year	15.4	8.0
All families	10.0	4.0

[a]These out-of-pocket expenses cover medical services; they do not include insurance premiums.
SOURCE: Medical Expenditure Panel Survey 1996 data across families of all sizes in Merlis, 2001.

threshold of out-of-pocket expenditures as were fully insured families in 1996 (Merlis, 2001; see Table 2.1). Paying medical bills can have profound, long-lasting economic and social effects on uninsured families (IOM, 2002b).

If the uninsured were to gain coverage, the change in their out-of-pocket costs would depend on both the scope of benefits and cost-sharing requirements.

What Are the Costs of Uncompensated Care Used by the Uninsured?

The best estimate of the value of *uncompensated health care* services provided to persons who lack health insurance for some or all of a year is roughly $35 billion annually, about 2.8 percent of total national spending for personal health care services (Hadley and Holahan, 2003b). This estimate includes the value of free hospital, physician, and clinic services that the uninsured use annually, adjusted to reflect spending in 2001.

About two-thirds of this uncompensated care ($23.6 billion) is public subsidies to hospitals, paid through federal Medicaid and Medicare *disproportionate share hospital (DSH) adjustments* and other financing mechanisms, state Medicaid DSH payments, and other state and local appropriations for the support of hospital services and operating costs. The public also supports a variety of governmental grant and direct care programs such as Community Health Centers, National Health Service Corps, Department of Veterans Affairs, and local health departments, amounting to about $7 billion annually. Donated physician time and services account for the remaining $5 billion of uncompensated care (Hadley and Holahan, 2003b).

If the uninsured were to gain coverage, some of the current spending for their health care would be redistributed among payers, for example, from physicians, who now provide uncompensated care, to taxpayers. Hospital bad debt and charity care caseloads would decline. As mentioned previously, the public sector already finances between 75 and 85 percent of the uncompensated care burden for uninsured individuals. Depending on the particular plan design, some of that amount could be reallocated to health insurance.

What Is the Cost of the Worse Health and Shorter Lives of Uninsured Americans?

In *Hidden Costs*, the Committee adapted an analytic strategy similar to that used by government agencies to estimate the benefits of life-saving and health-improving safety and environmental interventions in order to assess the economic losses borne by uninsured individuals as a result of their poorer health outcomes relative to those of insured counterparts. This analysis, commissioned by the Committee from economist Elizabeth Vigdor, is the first modeling exercise of its kind to evaluate the health benefits of coverage and is included in its entirety as Appendix B of *Hidden Costs* (2003b). Vigdor assigned an economic value to health by imputing a monetary value to a healthy life year and calculated the average difference in the present value in money terms of expected years of life in particular states of health between otherwise similar insured and uninsured populations. This difference constitutes an estimate of the economic value lost as a result of the current level of uninsurance within the U.S. population. Conversely, it is an estimate of the economic value of the better health outcomes that could be realized if the entire population had continuous health insurance coverage.

Based on this analysis, the Committee estimates that, in the aggregate, the diminished health and shorter life spans of Americans who lack health insurance are worth between $65 and $130 billion for each year spent without health insurance (IOM, 2003b). This estimate does not include *spillover* losses to families and society as a whole of the poorer health of the uninsured population. It does account for the value of those experiencing poorer health, including individual losses in work effort and developmental losses due to poor health in children. If the uninsured were to gain coverage comparable to that of the currently insured population, this $65–$130 billion in "*health capital*" would be an economic benefit rather than a cost.

The Committee's calculation of the economic value of improved health and longer life is likely an underestimate of the actual health benefits of continuous health insurance, in part because it only includes the effects up to age 65. Additional positive effects on health and longevity after age 65 also would be likely if health insurance were continuous before this age. In addition, there could be savings to the Medicare program. As it is now, there is likely to be pent-up demand for services at age 65 among those previously uninsured (IOM, 2003b).

Are Additional Costs Associated with Uninsurance?

Although the Committee could not develop specific dollar estimates, other public programs such as Social Security Disability Insurance and the criminal justice system likely have higher budgetary costs than they would if the U.S. population in its entirety had health insurance up to age 65 (IOM, 2003b).

Disability insurance claims could decrease with the health and functional status improvements that health insurance accords. Increased productivity in the workplace could also accompany increased population coverage rates. Studies have shown that productivity is lost on the job when workers have particular illnesses. Separate studies suggest that workers' health status can improve as a result of having coverage. However, the effects of coverage on workplace productivity have not been studied systematically or in any controlled fashion.

As already discussed above, persons with either private or public insurance are more likely than those without any coverage to receive appropriate treatment for mental health problems. More than 3 million adults have serious mental illness that can involve psychosis and aberrant behavior; 20 percent of these adults who do not reside in institutions lack health insurance. Between 600,000 and 700,000 persons with severe mental illness are jailed each year. Access to effective treatment prior to incarceration would be expected to reduce criminal justice expenses. Ironically, once people with serious mental illness have contact with the criminal justice system, they have an increased chance of obtaining access to specialty mental health services (McAlpine and Mechanic, 2000).

What Would the Additional Services Cost That the Uninsured Would Be Expected to Use if They Gained Coverage?

Closing the access gap for the uninsured would mean increased utilization of services. As described earlier, the uninsured population is less likely to use any kind of health service within a given year, and on average the uninsured person uses one-half to two-thirds of the volume and value of services that the privately insured person uses (IOM, 2003b). The Committee reviewed several sets of estimates of the value of the additional health services that would be provided to the uninsured once they became insured. Estimates of the additional costs of health services that the population that now lacks insurance could be expected to use if they gained coverage range from $34 billion to $69 billion a year in 2001 dollars. This range reflects the difference between the average per capita expenditure within public insurance programs (primarily Medicaid) and that for populations with private health insurance (Hadley and Holahan, 2003a). This range of estimated costs amounts to between 2.8 and 5.6 percent of national spending for personal health care services in 2001, equivalent to roughly half of the 8.7 percent increase in personal health care spending between 2000 and 2001 (IOM, 2003b).

These estimates do not reflect the costs of any particular plan to provide health insurance to the uninsured, nor do they include any costs of establishing a minimum benefit package that would affect the currently insured population. The cost range of $34 billion to $69 billion, which encompasses the results of three independent analyses, assumes no structural changes in the systems of health services delivery or finance, scope of benefits, or provider payment from those that currently operate in the public and private sectors (2003b). The defined benefit package for covering the uninsured would influence the nature of benefits offered to the currently insured. If it were a relatively generous package and there were no other structural changes, the costs of additional services would be greater than the $69 billion because of greater use by the currently insured as well as new utilization by the previously uninsured. Ultimately, the full cost of any reform will depend on the specific features of the approach taken, an estimate of which is beyond the scope of this report.

In its previous report, the Committee assessed the individual health and longevity benefits of continuous health insurance coverage for the uninsured population relative to the costs of providing this population with the kind and amount of health care used by comparable insured populations (IOM, 2003b). The Committee concluded that the economic value that would be gained in terms of better health outcomes among those now uninsured would likely exceed the incremental resource costs of providing the uninsured with the level of services now used, on average, by demographically similar people with either public or private coverage. In addition, the Committee's estimate of providing this "insured" level of health care services to those who now lack coverage compares favorably with other societal investments in improving health and extending life (IOM, 2003b).

EFFECTS OF THE STRUCTURE OF INSURANCE

The current amalgam of service arrangements and the mix of public and private insurance sources were not designed as an integrated system; rather, they have resulted from the aggregation, over time, of initiatives and developments in both the private and public sectors. A variety of factors related to the terms and structure of insurance affect eligibility for and affordability of insurance. Current insurance mechanisms and programs do not match the needs of all persons over time. Life-course and employment transitions, in particular, result in gaps in coverage (Kuttner and McLaughlin, 2003).

Coverage Gaps Associated with Employment-Based Coverage

Nearly two-thirds of all firms offer health benefits to their employees (66 percent), with offer rates ranging from 55 percent for small firms employing 3 to 9 workers to 98 percent for firms employing 200 or more workers

(Kaiser/HRET, 2003). Most employees take up the offer of coverage or obtain coverage through a family member's workplace health insurance plan. The link between health insurance and employment, however, creates many opportunities for loss of coverage. Job loss and retirement increase the risk of losing coverage. Work choices may be constrained for those with private coverage by the need to obtain and maintain health benefits with the current job (sometimes referred to as *job lock*). Even people who receive public insurance coverage may be limited in their job choices because of means testing for public benefits (IOM, 2002b).

Many of the uninsured, however, are not eligible for the plan offered where they work or work in settings that do not offer any plan. During the mid-1990s, only 55 percent of workers who earned less than $7 per hour were offered employment-based insurance compared with 96 percent of workers whose hourly rate was above $15 per hour (Cooper and Schone, 1997). This can result in inequities in coverage even if total family income is the same. A family having a single wage earner with a salary of $50,000 is more likely to have access to health insurance than is a family of two wage earners, each of whom earns an annual salary of $25,000.[8] So while working improves the chances of coverage, even members of families with two full-time wage earners have an 8 percent chance of being uninsured (Hoffman and Wang, 2003).

The prime economic force behind the declining portion of Americans covered by employment-based insurance is the gap between workers' purchasing power and increases in health services costs and costs of purchasing insurance (Cooper and Schone, 1997; Holahan and Kim, 2000; Cutler, 2002). In constant 1998 dollars, the cost of employment-based insurance increased 260 percent between 1977 and 1998 and the employee's share of insurance premiums increased 350 percent (Gabel, 1999). During the same period, median household incomes increased in real terms by 17 percent (U.S. Census Bureau, 2000). Health care cost increases exceeded growth in the general economy due to factors that included technology changes and increased use of services per capita, including prescription drugs (Glied, 2003). A recent econometric analysis by David Cutler (2002) concluded that virtually all of the decline in employee take-up rates between 1988 and 2001 (for full-time male workers, from 94 to 90 percent take-up of offers of coverage) could be attributed to increases in the employee share of premiums over this period.

---

[8]The distinction between the income of a "health insurance unit," i.e., family members who qualify for coverage together, and that of a household is important to the interpretation of coverage trends. For example, some have concluded that the increase of 1.4 million uninsured persons between 2000 and 2001 in the CPS represents an influx of middle-income persons, because about 800,000 of them lived in households with yearly incomes of at least $75,000 (Mills, 2002). Analyzing these estimates in terms of health insurance units, however, and accounting for changes in household composition supports a different conclusion: an increasing number of people with lower incomes joined households that earned over $75,000 annually, and almost all of the newly uninsured in 2001 (1.3 million people) were in families that earned less than twice the federal poverty level (Holahan, et al., 2003b).

Coverage Gaps Due to Differing Eligibility Rules for Members of the Same Family

Achieving coverage of the entire family can prove difficult (IOM, 2002b). Private insurers often restrict the definition of family to a traditional family structure. This mismatch between insurers' eligibility criteria and a functional family unit affects coverage. Most publicly financed health insurance programs are even more restrictive because they provide coverage for individuals rather than for families. Lower income parents are more likely to lack coverage than are their children because public programs provide coverage for children up to higher family income levels than they do for adults. Public programs also tend to have more generous family income limits for younger children than older ones, with the result that uninsurance rates are higher among older children (Hoffman and Wang, 2003).

Furthermore, simplification of eligibility rules and enrollment processes can reduce barriers to coverage. More than half of the 7.8 million children uninsured in 2002 were eligible for Medicaid or SCHIP coverage (Kenney et al., 2003). Parents' decisions on whether, when, and from whom to seek care for their children may be influenced by their own experiences with and knowledge of the health system (IOM, 2002b). When states have expanded Medicaid programs broadly to include low-income parents as well as their children, the enrollment of eligible children has increased more than it has in states without the broader parental coverage (Ku and Broaddus, 2000).

Gaps Because of the Cost of Coverage

The national average total annual premium for a family policy in an employment-based group exceeded $9,000 in 2003, with workers themselves picking up, on average, 27 percent of the cost of family coverage (Kaiser/HRET, 2003). In firms with at least 35 percent low-waged workers, employees pay a greater portion of the premium, typically 36 percent of the premium—an extra $68 per month compared with the national average (Kaiser/HRET, 2003). For a worker earning $20,000 per year, roughly $10 per hour, the employee's premium share for family coverage would take more than 16 percent of his or her income before taxes.

When it is available, individual coverage is often a stop-gap measure for adult children who lose their coverage as dependents before they can obtain job-based coverage and for retirees under the age of 65 before they become eligible for Medicare. A study comparing premiums for individual and group insurance plans with comparable benefits (comprehensive, preferred provider organization) in 17 health insurance markets found that for young adults (27 years old), the median premium for individually purchased (nongroup) coverage is roughly comparable to the premium for group coverage, especially for men, but that the median premium for individually purchased coverage for 55-year-olds is more than twice the premium for group coverage (Gabel et al., 2002).

Underwriting assumptions account for some of the differences in premiums that employers and employees face (IOM, 2001a). The price of an insurance premium that the insurer offers to a firm reflects a number of considerations, including firm size, whether it is unionized, the employment sector, and any risk or *experience rating* of the employees. Employers have sought ways to economize by increasing employee premiums and *cost sharing*, dropping coverage for retirees, and restricting benefit packages.

Gaps in Service Coverage and Their Effects

Lack of coverage affects the availability of care across the spectrum of preventive health services, chronic disease care, medications, mental health, acute care, emergency room treatment, and hospital care. When health insurance includes preventive and screening services, prescription drugs, and mental health care as well as acute and diagnostic care, it is more strongly associated with the receipt of appropriate care than when insurance does not have these features (IOM, 2002a).

Generally, insurance benefits are less likely to include preventive and screening services than physician visits for acute care or diagnostic tests for symptomatic conditions. A positive and statistically significant "dose-response" relationship has been found between the extent of coverage for preventive services and their receipt (Faulkner and Schauffler, 1997). Yet as long as people have some form of health insurance, even if it does not cover preventive services, they are more likely to receive appropriate services, partly because they are more likely to have a regular source of care or a primary provider (IOM, 2002a).

Adults with mental health coverage are more likely to receive mental health services from both general medical and specialty mental health providers and to receive care consistent with clinical practice guidelines than are those without any health insurance or with insurance that does not cover mental health conditions. Receipt of appropriate care has been associated with improved functional outcomes for depression and anxiety disorders (Sturm and Wells, 1995; Wang et al., 2000). Studies also show that uninsured adults with severe mental illnesses receive less appropriate care or medications and experience delays in receiving services until they gain insurance coverage (Rabinowitz et al., 1998, 2001; McAlpine and Mechanic, 2000).

Lack of insurance also can impede access to necessary prescription drugs. For example, persons without health insurance have been shown to wait an average of 4 months longer than privately insured patients to receive newer drug therapies for HIV (Shapiro et al., 1999). Only 43 percent of uninsured children have their prescriptions filled compared with 61 percent of privately insured and 56 percent of publicly insured children (McCormick et al., 2001).

SUMMARY

Health insurance is one of the most common, flexible, and reliable means used to gain access to health care. In the United States, health insurance is a voluntary matter, yet some people do not have the choice of coverage and many find it unaffordable. Because so many common events can precipitate the loss of insurance, the chance of being uninsured over the course of a lifetime is substantial. There is no guarantee for most people under the age of 65 that they will be eligible for or able to afford to purchase or retain health insurance. Reviewing the Committee's work to date allows us to draw some general conclusions important for designing effective strategies for extending coverage to everyone:

- Currently, health insurance coverage is not universal and it is not continuous, resulting in gaps in coverage that put people's health and finances at risk. Although coverage is needed throughout the course of life, persons can become uninsured regardless of age and family circumstances, with the notable exception of Medicare for those over age 65.
- Efforts to fill coverage gaps need to be affordable to individuals, employers, and the public budgets of government agencies that purchase insurance. Most uninsured families would need a substantial premium subsidy in order to purchase health insurance.
- Health insurance is important as a stable and efficiently targeted revenue source for health care service providers. Local communities with disproportionate populations without coverage are unable to shoulder the burden alone.
- Lack of coverage affects access to care across a spectrum of health care services. A high uninsured rate in a community can also affect availability of primary through tertiary care for both uninsured and insured community residents.
- Lack of coverage affects the amount and adequacy of care delivered and ultimately health outcomes. Having coverage for preventive health services, chronic disease care, medications, mental health, acute and diagnostic care, and hospital care promotes improved access to these services and improved health outcomes. Coverage increases the likelihood of receipt of cost-effective, evidence-based services in the appropriate settings (e.g., avoiding expensive crisis care for chronic conditions such as hypertension or asthma with regular use of appropriate ambulatory care). Increased coverage is especially likely to improve the health of people who are in the poorest health and who are most disadvantaged in terms of access to care and thus would likely reduce health disparities among racial and ethnic groups. Broad-based health insurance strategies across the entire uninsured population would be more likely to produce the desired health benefits than would "rescue" programs aimed only at the seriously ill or those continuing to piece together categorical coverage.

- Public dollars are not as well targeted to achieve improvements in health across the population as they could be if everyone had insurance-based financing for health care services.
- Current health insurance arrangements are complex and inefficient.
- When insurance becomes available, the uninsured will use more health services. Their increased use would be a positive change; the services, quality, and continuity of care that those without coverage do *not* get accounts for their poorer health outcomes compared with otherwise similar insured persons.
- Federal or shared federal-state health insurance programs distribute the burden of financing health care more broadly among taxpayers than the costs of uncompensated care, which fall more heavily on local communities with concentrations of uninsured residents. Insurance-based financing could alleviate some of the financial demands on communities disproportionately affected by uninsurance.

3

Eliminating Uninsurance: Lessons from the Past and Present

Despite nearly a century of efforts and incremental reforms to extend coverage, the nation's multiple sources of coverage leave 15 percent of the total population uninsured. This chapter develops the historical context of national reform efforts to reduce or eliminate uninsurance in the United States. It then looks at relatively recent federal initiatives to broaden coverage substantially and extension of coverage by some states and counties that have taken leadership roles. Past efforts offer useful lessons for reforming health care financing today.

Federal, state, and county reforms have not eliminated uninsurance, although some initiatives have improved access to health services or resulted in better health outcomes for populations who had lacked coverage. Some reforms have affected the basic structure of health care finance, while others have had a more limited focus, building on existing public programs or private insurance. The Committee's principles for assessing coverage proposals derive from the historical record as well as from its examination of the consequences of uninsurance.

NATIONAL EFFORTS TO BROADEN COVERAGE, 1916–1984

The lack of universal health insurance in the United States is in part a legacy of early twentieth-century precedents in the organization and financing of health services in the United States. It also reflects the absence of political leadership strong, broad, and sustained enough to forge a consensus in favor of universal coverage, despite public support, in the face of opposition from overlapping yet at times incompatible economic interests forged within the constraints of American political institutions and processes (Oberlander, 2003). Our government's federal structure and the independence of the legislative and executive branches place a relatively great burden on proponents of change.

Coverage reform first became a national issue in the early 1900s, when relatively few people had health insurance and most health care was purchased out of pocket or provided charitably. Over the next 70 years, a series of campaigns attempted to bring about greater coverage nationally. Early campaigns to create mandatory coverage were opposed by the medical profession, commercial insurers, and the business community. From the 1930s through the 1970s, the House Ways and Means Committee of the U.S. Congress determined the fate of most federal legislation to extend coverage, and most proposed reforms were prevented from coming before the full House for a vote.

In the context of the lack of federal legislation for more widespread public coverage, consumer demand fueled the rapid growth of private-sector coverage, starting in the mid-1930s. The nonprofit Blue Cross and Blue Shield plans, and subsequent plans from commercial insurers, enrolled millions of subscribers and by the early 1960s most Americans were insured through employment-based coverage. The enactment of the Medicare and Medicaid amendments to the Social Security Act in 1965 filled some of the gaps left by the emerging employment-based approach to financing care. Medicare extended coverage to most of the population over age 65 as well as to smaller groups of eligible persons (the permanently disabled). State implementation of the Medicaid program increased coverage significantly among categories of the low-income population. By the 1970s, the growth in total health care spending facilitated by the creation of Medicare made the issue of controlling health care spending and inflation central to universal coverage reform proposals. The early 1980s marked a high point for coverage levels nationally. Since that time, there has been a gradual increase in the number, and in most years the proportion, of uninsured persons under age 65. See Box 3.1 for a timeline of these efforts.

The sections that follow briefly review this history in order to illustrate important issues and basic tensions in the political sphere that have shaped more recent reform efforts. It is organized roughly chronologically, with diversions from the timeline to allow focus on specific topics.

Early Efforts: From Protecting the Income of Industrial Workers to Social Insurance for Improving Access to Care

Social insurance programs in late nineteenth-century Europe (for example, Germany, 1883) and Great Britain (1911) that included health insurance, and experience with the limited prepaid medical services available to fraternal or mutual benefit society members, spurred interest in universal coverage in the United States (Numbers, 1978). Initial organized efforts to extend coverage broadly occurred during the years around World War I (Starr, 1982). Early twentieth-century America was in the throes of rapid industrial and urban growth, with a booming population of low-income working families. With an eye toward allevi-

BOX 3.1
Landmarks in the History of Coverage

1916–1920   American Association for Labor Legislation campaigns for publicly administered, private-sector sickness insurance to protect the lost income of workers and their families

1932   Committee on the Costs of Medical Care final report calls for group organization and payment of health services on voluntary basis

1935   Social Security Act

1939   First of series of Wagner-Murray-Dingell bills in U.S. Congress that propose universal health insurance as social insurance

1942   War Labor Board ruling permits employers to exclude employment-based coverage from taxable income

1945   President Truman's "Fair Deal" proposal includes publicly financed and administered universal coverage

1948   U.S. Supreme Court ruling (Inland Steel) permits collective bargaining for employment-based coverage

1960   Social Security Act Amendments including Kerr-Mills program creating federal grants to the states to finance health services for poor persons at least 65 years of age (seniors)

1965   Social Security Act Amendments that create Medicare and Medicaid, nearly universal publicly and privately financed coverage for seniors and federally guaranteed eligibility for public coverage for specific categories of the poor

1971–1974   President Nixon and U.S. Congress introduce and debate proposals for universal coverage through a mix of public and private sources, fail to reach a vote in Congress

ating the economic burden of illness, a relatively small group of elite reformers, organized as the American Association for Labor Legislation (AALL), campaigned for mandatory workplace-based "sickness insurance." Sickness insurance, often called health insurance after the English precedent, was modeled after recently created state workmen's compensation programs (Numbers, 1978).[1] It targeted

---

[1]For example, former President Theodore Roosevelt made sickness insurance one of the planks in his ultimately unsuccessful campaign against Woodrow Wilson in 1912 on the Progressive ticket (Numbers, 1985).

1974	Employee Retirement Income Security Act, prohibiting state regulation of self-insured employer health plans.
1981	President Reagan's proposals to turn Medicaid into block grants to the states, in the Omnibus Budget Reconciliation Act of 1981
1984–1990	Expansions of Medicaid to pregnant women, infants, and children at higher income levels and delinking from eligibility for (state) income support
1985	Consolidated Omnibus Budget Reconciliation Act of 1985, with provision to improve continuity of employment-based coverage.
1993–1994	President Clinton's Health Security Act proposal for universal coverage through publicly administered, publicly and privately financed regional purchasing alliances created and debated, fails to reach a vote in Congress
1996	Federal welfare reform delinks Medicaid from income support programs, bars legal immigrants from Medicaid eligibility for first five years of residency
1996	Health Insurance Portabilitiy and Accountability Act, with provisions to improve continuity of coverage
1997	State Children's Health Insurance Program, extending public insurance eligibility to children in families earning between 100 and 200 percent of federal poverty level, expansions to their parents
2002	Trade Act, with provision for health insurance premium tax credit for groups of workers displaced by international commerce and retirees

industrial workers and their families and included a cash benefit to replace lost income, access to free health care, and a death benefit; premiums would be paid by employers, workers, and the state (Starr, 1982; Hoffman, 2001). The plan was not universal, for it excluded most African Americans and other ethnic minorities by not including agricultural, domestic, and temporary workers. In addition, it restricted eligibility to employed men and women earning less than $1,200 annually (low income but not poor), assuming that the poor could rely on charity and that the middle class could afford to purchase their own care (Hoffman, 2001).

Between 1916 and 1920, the AALL's model sickness insurance bill was debated in a number of state legislatures in more urban and industrial parts of the United States, most notably California and New York, with support from many governors and state-level fact-finding commissions (Numbers, 1978; Hoffman, 2001). Ultimately, these bills were defeated. Key opponents included:

- the American Medical Association (AMA), an early supporter that became an outspoken opponent as rank-and-file members (county medical societies), gaining experience with contract practice under the new workmen's compensation programs, grew concerned that insurance would interfere with the practice of medicine and threaten the economic viability of solo practice;
- employers who did not welcome broadened financial responsibility for the health of their workforce and who predicted higher costs passed along to consumers and the loss of jobs;
- commercial insurers who stood to lose their lucrative business selling death benefits (industrial insurance) to low-income workers and who were excluded from the proposed state-level administration of sickness insurance; and
- organized labor, principally Samuel Gompers of the American Federation of Labor, to whom mandatory coverage was a threat to the organizing ability of unions (Numbers, 1978; Starr, 1982; Hoffman, 2001).

Proposals for state sickness insurance programs were abandoned by 1920, felled by the lack of political leadership, the difficulties of enacting mandatory policies on a state-by-state basis, and the AALL's inability to build coalitions and fashion workable political compromises with the economic interests that opposed its model for expanding health insurance (Numbers, 1985). In addition, a harmful legacy of this first political battle was the framing of mandated coverage as counter to American values, with coverage proposals attacked in newspapers and speeches as fundamentally Germanic, and, after the close of World War One and the onset of the Red Scare, as expressions of Bolshevism (Hoffman, 2001).
Starting in the 1920s, demand for health care services by the middle class, fed by the improved effectiveness of hospital-based care and the increasing risk of high-cost medical expenses, reinvigorated public debate about extending coverage (Starr, 1982; Stevens, 1989). Unlike the sickness insurance proposals of the 1910s, the goals of reform were to increase utilization, and health care spending, by making care and coverage more affordable to all Americans universally, not only low-income workers and their dependents (Starr, 1982; Derickson, 2002).
During the 1930s and into the 1940s, proposals to extend public coverage significantly took the form of social insurance for all Americans, resembling the system of federal pensions created by the Social Security Act of 1935. Proposed reforms drew on the work of an independent group of scholars and physicians, the Committee on the Costs of Medical Care, that advocated both group practice and financing for care, to rationalize health services delivery and make health care

more affordable (Starr, 1982). Because much domestic policy making for the nation now took place at the federal rather than the state level, health finance reformers faced a number of new challenges, including the separation of powers (so that Presidential support would not necessarily be matched by congressional support); a lack of party discipline within the two houses of Congress; powerful regional voting blocks and interest group lobbies; and the ideological constraints of single-party reform efforts (Marmor, 1973; Maioni, 1998).

In the 1930s, organized labor supported a publicly mandated extension of coverage, but the medical profession, insurance industry, and business interests continued to resist such proposals. The AMA in particular was a strong political presence in Washington, and its vigorous lobbying of Congress and the public in favor of voluntary rather than mandatory coverage threatened the passage of New Deal legislation, and the President's bid for reelection. In response, President Franklin Roosevelt's Administration cut a provision for health insurance from what became the Social Security Act of 1935 (Marmor, 1973; Starr, 1982; Maioni, 1998). In an effort to revive universal coverage proposals, which many perceived as the "missing piece" of the New Deal, in 1939 reform-minded members of Congress began introducing universal coverage bills each year (labeled Wagner-Murray-Dingell bills, after their key sponsors) that framed coverage as a means to lower financial barriers, made eligibility universal (not only for persons in the Social Security system), and included grants-in-aid to the states to support indigent care (Maioni, 1998). None of these bills was reported out of the Ways and Means Committee, undone by the lack of leadership by President Roosevelt and the slim voting majority of the Democrats in Congress that was insufficient to pass controversial reform (Marmor, 1973; Maioni, 1998).

Universal coverage bills stalled in Congress, but consumer demand for health insurance grew. While commercial insurers were slow to enter the market for group policies organized through the workplace, nonprofit and independent organizations created prepayment plans for hospital services, indemnity and service benefit plans for physician care, and sites for the direct delivery of services that gave fundamental shape to the organization and financing of health services in subsequent decades. The locally organized and directed Blue Cross hospitalization plans and Blue Shield physician plans expanded rapidly from their origins in the early 1930s to become the single largest source of coverage by the 1950s (Cunningham and Cunningham, 1997). Community organizations such as Group Health Cooperative of Puget Sound, consumer cooperatives and private clinics, and health plans organized around industries, such as Kaiser Permanente, extended both coverage and services (Somers and Somers, 1961; Starr, 1982). Enrollment of workers and their dependents in private coverage soared: between 1940 and 1960, the proportion of the general population with private coverage grew from 9.1 percent (about 12 million people) to 67.8 percent (about 122 million people) (Etheredge, 1990; Bovbjerg et al., 1993). Offering health insurance as a benefit was attractive to employers, given the exemption from federal taxes of the employers' contributions to health insurance premiums (codified in the Internal Review Code of 1954) (Starr, 1982).[2]

Although private-sector coverage grew quickly, there was continued public and legislative interest in universal health insurance. After World War II, the federal government's role in many aspects of health policy expanded, for example, in the funding of biomedical research and hospital construction, but congressional resistance, bolstered by the lobbying of reform opponents, blocked public mandates for coverage (Marmor, 1973; Fox, 1986). The first president to champion universal coverage, Harry Truman revisited this issue in the late 1940s, fighting a contentious political battle against the AMA, commercial insurers, and the business community in a failed bid to convince the 80th and 81st Congresses to enact Wagner-Murray-Dingell legislation (Starr, 1982).[3] President Truman added the key ingredient of political leadership but lacked sufficient votes in Congress, facing a hostile reception in Congress from Southern Democrats committed to reversing New Deal policies and opposed to his Administration's civil rights policies (Poen, 1979; Maioni, 1998). The only public coverage to be expanded would be federal grants-in-aid to the states to support indigent care, in the 1950 Amendments to the Social Security Act (Stevens, 1989).

In the 1950s enrollment in commercial policies outgrew that of nonprofits (Somers and Somers, 1961; Starr, 1982; Cunningham and Cunningham 1997). One advantage that commercial insurers could offer purchasers of group policies was a less expensive alternative to nonprofit "community rating" (where actuarial risk was spread broadly through uniform premiums) in the form of "experience-rating," or charging premiums according to the claims experience of the employer's workforce. Experience rating made policies less expensive for healthier employee groups and more expensive or unavailable for individuals, particularly ill or disabled persons, who tried to purchase coverage outside the workplace (Starr, 1982). The growing centrality of health insurance revenue to the fiscal health of the health care system created interest on the part of providers (physicians, hospitals) in seeing greater numbers of the general population covered by insurance, albeit on a voluntary basis (IOM, 2003a). For persons without coverage, the price of being uninsured was growing, as the increasingly widespread coverage fueled higher costs for health care and doubled hospital prices during the 1950s (Starr, 1982).

Following the defeat of President Truman's campaign for universal coverage

---

[2]In 1942, a War Labor Board ruling made health coverage an attractive fringe benefit for employers to offer workers, whose salaries were restricted due to wartime wage controls; between 1942 and 1945, there was more than a fourfold increase in group hospitalization enrollment (Starr, 1982). A 1948 U.S. Supreme Court decision allowed unions to collectively bargain for health insurance, and enrollment jumped (Starr, 1982; Gabel, 1999).

[3]The Truman Administration's proposal included medical and hospital benefits and federal grants-in-aid to the states to finance premiums for the poor, with national administration and financing through a 3 percent payroll tax split between firms and workers (Marmor, 1973).

in the late 1940s, proposals to extend health insurance by means of public policies focused on incremental change. In 1951, the handful of public officials who had worked for universal coverage shifted tactics, proposing a new 60-day hospitalization benefit for Social Security beneficiaries. This benefit would be funded off-budget, using Social Security trust dollars to lessen the economic burden of health services already used by the over-65 population (rather than to increase access to care) who were less likely to carry private insurance (Maioni, 1998). Their proposal aided the perception that the middle class (i.e., those who had paid Social Security taxes) had earned such coverage. They sidestepped AMA criticism by not including physician services (Marmor, 1973).[4] The proposed reform brought out traditional allies and opponents of mandatory coverage extensions, pitting the AMA against organized labor (the AFL-CIO) (Starr, 1982). Annual hearings on hospitalization proposals failed to advance reform, although the 1960 Kerr-Mills Act amending Social Security did acknowledge the interest in financing care for low-income seniors, increasing grants-in-aid to the states that raised sufficient matching funds (Marmor, 1973).

An Incremental Compromise for Universal Coverage: Medicare and Medicaid

In the late 1950s, the level of health insurance coverage was at an all-time high, although only about 8 percent of the population had coverage that could be called comprehensive (i.e., insurance that covered hospital stays and physician services) (Somers and Somers, 1961). Employment-based coverage was becoming the norm, with gaps of uninsured populations growing among those who did not or could not receive an employer's offer of group coverage.

A crescendo of political and legislative activity on hospital insurance in the early 1960s led to the first significant extension of publicly mandated coverage (Medicare and Medicaid) after the 1964 elections returned President Lyndon B. Johnson to the White House and brought large Democratic majorities favoring passage to Congress. In the years immediately before, President John F. Kennedy had campaigned for a Social Security hospitalization benefit, a scaled-down approach compared with President Truman's universal coverage proposals.

Despite annual hearings, the garnering of public support by the Administration, and the strategic building of votes on the Hill, House Ways and Means Chair Wilbur Mills released a coverage bill only after legislative developments in 1964 and the elections threatened his continued leadership on health insurance (Marmor, 1973; Maioni, 1998). When the 89th Congress convened in 1965, Medicare was

---

[4]Proposals tied to the Social Security system were not for universal coverage; in 1952, only 7 million of the roughly 12.5 million persons over age 65 would have been covered by the proposed reform (Marmor, 1973).

at the top of the agenda and was signed into law later that year, together with Medicaid, as amendments to the Social Security Act (Fox, 1986; Hacker, 1997). Medicare and Medicaid passed because of the unique legislative alignments of 1965 and also because of Chairman Mills' leadership in crafting a political compromise acceptable to interest groups, especially the AMA, which continued to lobby against the Administration's plans (Marmor, 1973; Maioni, 1998). He described the amendments as a "three-layer cake" with something for everyone:

- Medicare—consisting of Part A, hospitalization, for which there is automatic and permanent enrollment and financing through Social Security, and Part B, coverage for physician visits, with voluntary one-time enrollment and a monthly premium payment—provided nearly universal coverage for persons ages 65 and older.[5] Part A achieved the goal of social insurance advocates and the Johnson Administration, while Part B accommodated the AMA's objections to a mandatory program.
- Medicaid, the third layer of the cake, covers certain categories of low-income persons and makes existing grants-in-aid to state programs more uniform in terms of eligibility and benefits (Marmor, 1973).[6] Medicaid addressed the interest of the hospital industry in alleviating the burden of uncompensated care.

To win support for passage from provider groups, the new law essentially adopted the reimbursement approaches of Blue Shield (for physicians) and Blue Cross (for hospitals), including few limits on reimbursement for physicians, and added favorable provisions to pay hospitals for capital depreciation. However, these two aspects of the 1965 statute laid the groundwork for significant growth in health care inflation and spending (Starr, 1982).[7]

The Medicare and Medicaid Amendments represented a limited extension of health insurance coverage. Medicare also augured for improved access to care for African Americans, as certification for a hospital to participate in the program was conditioned on its desegregated status (Reynolds, 1997). While social insurance advocates saw the amendments as an opening wedge for future growth in coverage levels, more pragmatic observers interpreted their design as a way to fend off

---

[5]Amendments have added Medicare coverage for persons certified to be permanently and totally disabled and persons with end-stage renal disease (IOM, 2001a).

[6]Eligibility to enroll in Medicaid involves fulfilling requirements related to income and assets (making it a so-called means-tested program) and being a member of a specific group or category that is eligible for benefits, for example, a minor child. Those who meet economic and categorical criteria must also meet immigration status and state residency requirements. Eligibility standards vary by state and have changed from year to year, with general oversight provided by the federal government (IOM, 2001a).

[7]The Hill Burton Act of 1946 substantially expanded hospital capacity across the nation in the years before implementation of Medicare, contributing to the availability and utilization of health services nationally.

further broadening of the public mandate. For example, financing Medicare physician services with general tax revenues and beneficiary contributions, and using Medicaid to fill coverage gaps for persons under age 65, extended coverage while reinforcing existing approaches (i.e., voluntary coverage for the services most often used, and means-testing for benefits for the poor) (Marmor, 1973).

Implementation of Medicare and Medicaid introduced tens of millions of newly insured persons, and billions of new public dollars, into the health care system. By 1970, 20.5 million people were enrolled in Medicare and 18 million people in Medicaid (Bovbjerg et al., 1993). Between 1965 and 1975, annual federal spending on health care jumped from less than $10 billion to more than $40 billion (Hacker, 1997). There was a dramatic increase in utilization; within a year of implementation, 20 percent of all persons 65 years and older had used Medicare for hospital services and 12 million had used Part B coverage for physician services (Marmor, 1973). Nevertheless, gaps in coverage and financial protection remained. Medicaid covered only an estimated one-third of those considered poor, and Medicare reimbursed less than half of seniors' spending on health and long-term care services (Starr, 1982).

Paying for Reform: Cost Containment Joins Access as a Focus for Reform in the Years Since 1965

With federal taxes supporting coverage for a large segment of the population, and with the country in an economic recession, the rapidly increasing costs of health care to society overall and interest in improving the efficiency (including financing) of the health care system motivated reform (Starr, 1982; Lewis, 1983; Steinmo and Watts, 1995; Hacker, 1997). Public officials, insurers, and employers were united in the widely shared belief that a poorly organized and inefficient health care system fueled health care inflation and that universally mandated coverage could bring cost savings (Starr, 1982).[8] A combination of factors defeated efforts to extend coverage further. Some were unique to the political circumstances of the day (i.e., the impeachment proceedings against President Nixon and Wilbur Mills' fall from power in 1974). Others, such as the inability to fashion a workable consensus on a congressional bill and opposition from commercial insurers and employers, were familiar from earlier efforts to achieve broad-based reforms. As analyst Stuart Altman has observed of the era, which leads up to the present, many policy actors who previously opposed reform altogether have joined the call for change, but they have often been unwilling to compromise their own vision of reform and the absence of change has been the second-best or fallback option (Kahn and Pollack, 2001).

During the early 1970s, members of Congress and the Nixon Administration

---

[8]Such interest in improving the design and efficiency of the health care system was reflected in the Health Maintenance Organization Act of 1973, for example.

generated a number of bills to extend coverage and constrain costs, either by filling gaps in the existing mix of public and private coverage (the Nixon Administration's proposed employer mandate funded by a payroll tax, paired with expanded public coverage and regulation of payment rates) or by replacing privately purchased policies with a federally administered system under a national budget (e.g., Senator Edward Kennedy's Health Security Act of 1970) (Starr, 1982; Etheredge, 1990; Hacker, 1997; Maioni, 1998). Despite the resistance of providers, employers (especially small businesses), insurers, and the states to the regulatory aspects of proposed reform, passage of a universal coverage bill came close in 1974 (Starr, 1982; Etheredge, 1990; Steinmo and Watts, 1995; Hacker, 1997). President Nixon's February message to Congress laid out a Comprehensive Health Insurance Plan that combined Medicare, Medicaid, and an employer mandate (Davis, 2001). The lack of political leadership to forge a consensus on one of the many proposed plans in Congress by the summer of 1974, however, combined with the turmoil of President Nixon's August resignation and the decision of organized labor to withhold its support from reform until after the November elections, resulted in the disintegration of what bipartisan agreement existed (Starr, 1982; Maioni, 1998). After 1974, ongoing economic recession and price inflation, particularly in health care, sank any further serious debate about reforming health care financing to extend coverage. Cost controls became the key emphasis during the Ford and Carter Administrations.[9]

By the late 1970s, health insurance coverage reached its highest level yet; in 1980, roughly 15 percent of the general population under age 65 was uninsured, about 29.6 million people (Bovbjerg et al., 1993). From 1970 to 1980, aggregate spending on health care had continued to grow, from $69 billion to $230 billion and from 7.2 percent to 9.4 percent of the gross domestic product (Starr, 1982). For employers, health insurance premiums were becoming more expensive, leading them to increase deductibles, decrease dependent coverage, and, as the 1980s wore on, turn to commercial managed care contracting to restrain health care cost increases (Hacker, 1997). In an effort to restrain the continued growth of health care spending under Medicare, federal officials replaced fee-for-service reimbursement with capitation. During the 1980s, there would be incremental public expansions, particularly through the Medicaid program, which will be discussed later in this chapter. Absent major reforms of health care financing to extend coverage in the future, the stage was set for the major increases in the number of uninsured seen during the 1980s (Lewis, 1983; Hacker, 1997).

Interest in comprehensive national reform of health care financing surfaced again in the early 1990s. Economic recession and continuing health care inflation renewed interest among middle-class voters (Hacker, 1997). During President

---

[9]The Carter Administration did develop a universal coverage proposal, never introduced in Congress, called the National Health Plan, which divided coverage between private sources (employer mandate) and public sources (a federal program to replace Medicare and Medicaid and expand eligibility to all lower income persons) (*Congressional Quarterly*, 1977; Davis, 2001).

Clinton's first term, his Administration convened a task force of hundreds of experts to craft a legislative proposal for universal coverage (Hoffman, 2001). The Clinton plan was built around an employer mandate, and within the confines of a large federal deficit, with the federal government both restraining health care costs and extending coverage through regional purchasing pools (Skocpol, 1996; Hacker, 1997). Private managed care health plans would compete for contracts with the regional pools, introducing the idea of managed competition (Enthoven, 1978a,b; Starr, 1992; Hacker, 1997). Although there is no single definitive explanation for the failure to enact universal coverage in the mid-1990s, many analytic interpretations stress the Administration's difficulties in mobilizing public and political support for the complex proposal, the uncertainties involved in the proposed overhaul of the nation's health care financing and delivery arrangements, and the crystallization of Republican opposition to the Clinton proposal as contributing to the defeat of the plan before it reached a vote in Congress (Skocpol, 1996; Hacker, 1997; Marmor and Barer, 1997). There was vigorous political opposition of provider, insurer, and business community groups, many of whom favored reform but perceived the terms of the Clinton proposal to be economically threatening. This opposition played out in media campaigns that lowered public support for proposed reform.

Despite multiple reform campaigns over the past century, enduring characteristics have shaped the current fragmented approach to financing health care services, including:

- **the presence of well-organized and well-financed provider, insurer, and business groups with economic stakes potentially adversely affected by proposed coverage expansions (although many have agreed with the need for reform);**
- **the obstacles posed to comprehensive policy change by the American political process; and**
- **insufficient political leadership to fashion a workable consensus and then shepherd that consensus through the legislative process.**

In the wake of the failure to implement universal coverage, the federal, state, and some local governments in recent years have experimented with incremental coverage expansions with impacts much more modest than that of Medicare and Medicaid in the 1960s. In the sections that follow, the Committee will first explore federal expansions of Medicaid, the State Children's Health Insurance Program (SCHIP), and targeted federal programs related to employment-based coverage. Following that is a discussion of five states (Hawaii, Massachusetts, Minnesota, Oregon, and Tennessee) that have led the way in covering more residents. Lastly, the experiences of three counties that have adopted innovative approaches to extending coverage are discussed to illustrate local reform efforts and their limits.

FEDERAL INITIATIVES TO EXTEND COVERAGE SINCE 1984

The level of employment-based coverage has a fundamental effect on uninsurance. Public extensions of coverage at the federal, state, and local level, as well as public policies affecting the availability of individually purchased (nongroup) policies, have filled some of the gaps remaining from the employment-based approach (IOM, 2001a). Almost two-thirds of those under age 65 obtain health insurance through their workplace or that of a family member, with public programs covering an additional 15 percent and individually purchased policies almost 7 percent (Fronstin, 2002).

This section reviews major federal extensions of coverage since the mid-1980s, both public (Medicaid expansions to cover pregnant women, infants, and young children, and the State Children's Health Insurance Program) and private (federal regulation of the market for private insurance). None has approached even the partial success of the initial Medicare and Medicaid programs in boosting coverage in the general population. As Figure 3.1 depicts, there has been little overall change in the proportions of privately and publicly insured persons and in uninsured rate overall for the nation over the period from 1987 to 2002. Since the early 1980s, the number of uninsured persons under age 65 has grown in step with general population growth, while employment-based coverage has alternately grown, declined (in the late 1980s and early 1990s), grown again through the late 1990s, and has declined once again since the turn of the century. Tempered by public expansions of coverage, the uninsured rate as a result has varied within a few percentage points, between 14.9 percent and 17.2 percent of the noninstitutionalized population under age 65 (Levit et al., 1992; Fronstin, 2002; Mills and Bhandari, 2003).

Federal extensions of public coverage since the mid-1980s have often followed the lead of successful state insurance reforms, for example, in the case of SCHIP and the regulation of private-sector plans through the Health Insurance Portability and Accountability Act of 1996 (HIPAA) and the Consolidated Omnibus Budget Reconciliation Act of 1985 (COBRA). They have lowered uninsured rates among lower income children (in households earning less than 200 percent of poverty) and boosted the numbers of lower income persons with public coverage. At the same time, the proportion of adults with public coverage has declined, reflecting shifts in the demographic composition of the general population as well as public policy changes such as welfare reform. Concurrently with broadened eligibility for public coverage, new federal statutes (i.e., COBRA, HIPAA, and the Trade Act) have been enacted to protect and support the retention of workplace health benefits. These have established important precedents in principle for uninterrupted health insurance coverage but overall have had a limited impact on uninsurance, for reasons to be discussed.

These extensions have succeeded in improving coverage among selected groups when the programs receive adequate and stable public funding (particularly

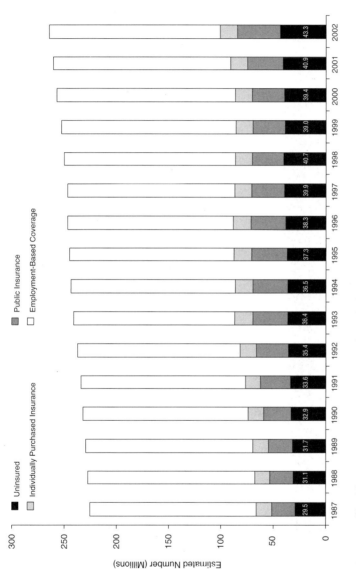

FIGURE 3.1 Sources of health insurance coverage and number of uninsured persons for population under age 65 years, 1987–2002.

NOTE: Coverage reported as military (i.e., Tricare, CHAMPVA) is counted as employment-based. Estimates for 2000, 2001, and 2002 use Census 2000-based weights. Precise estimates do not add to 100 percent due to rounding and because respondents may report more than one source of coverage within a year.

SOURCES: Fronstin, 2002; Mills and Bhandari, 2003.

federal dollars), when they foster continuity of coverage within families or among health plans, and when they make insurance coverage affordable both to individuals and families and to society over time. In addition to specific Committee findings for each of the expansions, to be discussed, the Committee draws three more general findings about federal initiatives.

Finding: Federal incremental reforms over the past 20 years have made little progress in reducing overall uninsured rates nationally, although public program expansions have improved coverage for targeted, previously uninsured groups. Federal reforms of employment-based insurance have not included provisions for assuring affordability and, thus, have had limited effect.

Finding: Extensions of program eligibility for one group of uninsured often affect the coverage status of other population groups indirectly, for example, when SCHIP enrollment efforts identify children who are eligible for but not enrolled in the Medicaid program.

Finding: Public programs fall short of their coverage goals when not all eligible persons enroll. When outreach and enrollment are made a priority, coverage levels rise. Public coverage programs sometimes employ administrative barriers to enrollment to contend with inadequate or unstable funding during periods of economic stress within the state.

Medicaid Expansions for Pregnant Women, Infants, and Children, 1984–1990

Finding: Incremental coverage extensions through Medicaid have been less effective than initially anticipated. A sizable population is eligible but not enrolled or does not maintain enrollment over time, diminishing the effectiveness of the coverage.

When Medicaid was created in 1965, some envisioned that Medicaid and Medicare together would fill the coverage gaps left by the employment-based health insurance system (Marmor, 1973). However, with categorical structures of eligibility tied to the rules of the cash assistance programs, the income eligibility levels then in existence, and funding shortfalls, state Medicaid programs did not cover all those with incomes too low to afford private health insurance coverage (Starr, 1982; Stevens, 1989).[10] Medicaid significantly raised the level of federal

---

[10]Most Medicaid enrollees have been low-income children and their mothers. A sizable group of adults are eligible for but not enrolled in Medicaid, roughly 16 percent of the 19 million uninsured

support for the states, with matching dollars pegged to per capita income in each state, and made eligibility for public coverage an entitlement. Such entitlement was limited to certain categories of persons (see Box 3.2 for current federal eligibility requirements); then, as now, single, childless adults under age 65 often are the group least eligible for Medicaid. The scope of each state's program dictates how far dollars go to pay for the federally mandated minimum benefits package for Medicaid recipients.

Expansion of the Medicaid program was prompted by public concern about the worsening health status of poor children, indicated by a reversal in the long-term decline in infant mortality rates, and the diminishing percentage of low-income children and mothers enrolled (due to more stringent eligibility standards for welfare) (Schlesinger and Kronebusch, 1990). Between 1984 and 1990, the Congress altered categorical eligibility requirements and gradually increased Medicaid income eligibility levels for pregnant women, infants, and children through provisions in its annual spending bills; Box 3.3 summarizes the legislative provisions. These changes delinked Medicaid coverage for pregnant women, infants, and children from the requirement that they meet their state's welfare eligibility requirements, a process continued with welfare reform in 1996 (KCMU, 2002a).[11]

Some states folded these changes into Section 1115 Medicaid waivers granted by the federal government for research and demonstration projects that are designed to be cost neutral. These and other waivers from required minimum benefits and restrictions on categories of eligibility allow states to offer coverage more widely within the limits of their federal matching funds (Lambrew, 2001). Under waivers, some states have reallocated Medicaid Disproportionate Share Hospital (DSH) funds to expand eligibility (e.g., Tennessee), while others have attempted to stretch Medicaid dollars by shifting portions of their Medicaid population from fee-for-service to managed care contracting (e.g., Arizona, Maryland, New York, and Rhode Island) or by dampening utilization by charging premiums

---

adults with incomes under twice the poverty level (Schneider, 2002). As of 2002, there were 47.2 million persons enrolled. More than half (51 percent) were children, about one-fifth (22 percent) were nondisabled adults under age 65, 17 percent were certified as blind or disabled, and another 10 percent were low-income persons at least 65 years old (KCMU, 2003b). The bulk of Medicaid's $212 billion spending goes for its blind and disabled recipients (44 percent of spending) and seniors (27 percent of spending). Children and nondisabled adults under age 65 together account for less than one-third of program spending (29 percent), though they represent 73 percent of enrollees.

[11]Through section 1931, part of the Personal Responsibility and Work Opportunity Reconciliation Act of 1996, Medicaid eligibility for parents was broadened, delinking Medicaid enrollment from welfare participation and basing minimum eligibility on a state's welfare eligibility criteria as of July 1996, even if parents were not enrolled in welfare. It also permitted states to loosen income and asset tests, as well as adjust these tests for inflation (so-called income and asset disregards) (Birnbaum, 2000; Broaddus et al., 2002).

BOX 3.2
Eligibility for Medicaid

The federal government requires that the following groups be entitled to enroll in Medicaid:

• federal required minimum: children under age 6 and pregnant women whose family income is below 133 percent of the federal poverty level (FPL) ($20,296 for a family of three in 2003);
• federal required minimum: children ages 6–18 with family incomes at or below 100 percent of FPL ($15,260 for a family of three in 2003);
• no federal minimum: states set income standards for adults without children; parents of children are categorically eligible if they meet income and asset tests. On average, the states' income eligibility level for parents is 41 percent of FPL ($6,257 for a family of three in 2003), varying from a low of 21 percent ($3,205 for a family of three) in Alabama to a high of 275 percent ($41,965 for a family of three) in Minnesota;
• Supplementary Security Income (SSI) recipients or those aged, blind, and disabled individuals who qualify in states that apply more restrictive eligibility requirements;
• recipients of adoption assistance and foster care who are under Title IV-E of the Social Security Act;
• special protected groups (typically individuals who lose their cash assistance from SSI due to earnings from work or increased Social Security benefits but may keep Medicaid for a period of time); and
• qualified Medicare beneficiaries, specified low-income Medicare beneficiaries, and disabled-and-working individuals who previously qualified for Medicare but lost their coverage because of their return to work.

and imposing cost sharing for new categories of enrollees (e.g., Arkansas, New Mexico, and Oregon) (Mann, 2002; Schneider, 2002).[12]

Expanding Medicaid eligibility levels brought concern that increased enrollment reflected the substitution of public insurance for employment-based coverage for workers and dependents at the lower end of the wage scale. Studies give a wide range of estimates of the amount of substitution (often referred to as "crowd out"), although none is fully comparable in terms of methods, data sources, or criteria measured (Cutler and Gruber, 1997; Dubay, 1999; Alteras, 2001). Early estimates of Medicaid substitution approaching 50 percent (Cutler and Gruber, 1996a, b) have since been reevaluated. Recent estimates have been as low as 4 percent, with upper bounds between 17 percent and 23 percent, depending on how substitution is defined and measured (Cutler and Gruber, 1997; Alteras, 2001). This concern about substitution of Medicaid coverage for employment-

---

[12]In 1997, federal law was revised so that implementation of Medicaid mandatory managed care contracting no longer required a Section 1115 waiver (Mann, 2002).

In addition, federal law permits the states to extend eligibility beyond the minimum requirements listed. Most but not all state expansions may be supported by federal matching funds. The most common optional expansions by the states including eligibility for the following groups:

- infants up to age 1 and pregnant women not covered under the mandatory rules whose family income is up to 185 percent of FPL;
- recipients of state supplementary income payments;
- certain aged, blind, or disabled adults who have incomes above those requiring mandatory coverage but below the FPL;
- persons receiving care under home and community-based waivers;
- persons infected with tuberculosis (TB) who would be financially eligible for Medicaid at the SSI income level (eligibility is only for TB-related ambulatory services and for TB drugs);
- institutionalized individuals with income and resources below specified limits;
- medically needy—persons who meet categorical requirements and have significant health care expenses with incomes in excess of the mandatory or optional levels; these individuals may "spend down" to Medicaid eligibility by incurring medical and/or remedial care expenses to offset their excess income, thus reducing it to a level below the maximum income allowed by that state's Medicaid plan; and
- legal resident aliens and other qualified aliens who entered the United States on or after August 22, 1996, made ineligible for Medicaid for five years because of the 1996 welfare reform law.

SOURCES: Broaddus et al., 2002; IOM, 2002b; KCMU, 2002b; DHHS, 2003.

sponsored health insurance, which influenced the design for SCHIP, will be discussed.

Infant mortality rates improved in the latter half of the 1980s, reflecting the development of neonatal intensive care units made possible by Medicaid financing even before the eligibility expansions (Cutler and Gruber, 1996b; Howell, 2001). One study estimates an 8.5 percent decrease in the infant mortality rate associated with the 30 percentage point increase in Medicaid eligibility for women of reproductive age (15 to 44 years old) between 1979 and 1992, with the expansions targeted to women eligible for welfare having more of an effect on health (Currie and Gruber, 1996b).

Millions of children and adults remain eligible for but not enrolled in Medicaid. Difficulties in enrolling and maintaining enrollment, confusion about eligibility, the decision by some who are eligible not to participate in public coverage, and, in the case of children, the diminished likelihood of enrollment when their parents are ineligible for the same program as their child, are uninsured or have weak connections to the health care system, all contribute to low take-up rates for Medicaid (IOM, 2002b; Schneider, 2002). Particularly for those at the upper end

BOX 3.3
Medicaid Expansions, 1984–1990

• **Deficit Reduction Act of 1984.** Medicaid eligibility required for children born after September 30, 1983, up to their fifth birthday, and for women either pregnant for the first time or pregnant in an unemployed family with two parents, in families eligible for Aid to Families with Dependent Children (AFDC) (welfare), roughly 40 percent of the FPL. Required eligibility for one year for infants born to Medicaid-eligible women.

• **Consolidated Omnibus Budget Reconciliation Act of 1985 (COBRA).** Medicaid eligibility required for children up to age 5 in families eligible for AFDC and for pregnant women in families both eligible for AFDC and with two parents (no longer required to be unemployed).

• **Omnibus Budget Reconciliation Act of 1986.** Option to expand Medicaid eligibility to pregnant women and children under age 5 in families earning no more than 100 percent FPL. Note that at the time, eligibility for state welfare programs averaged about 45 percent (KCMU, 2002a). Option to use presumptive and continuous eligibility to expand Medicaid to pregnant women.

• **Omnibus Budget Reconciliation Act of 1987.** Medicaid eligibility required for children under age 8 in families eligible for AFDC on basis of income. Option to expand Medicaid eligibility to pregnant women and infants in families earning no more than 185 percent of FPL and children under age 8 in families earning no more than 100 percent of FPL.

• **Medicare Catastrophic Coverage Act of 1988.** Medicaid eligibility required for pregnant women and infants in families earning less than 100 percent of FPL, to be implemented over time. Although most provisions of the Act were repealed in 1989, this provision remains in effect.

• **Family Support Act of 1988.** Option to expand Medicaid eligibility to pregnant women and children above required levels.

• **Omnibus Budget Reconciliation Act of 1989.** Medicaid eligibility required for pregnant women and children under age 6 in families earning no more than 133 percent of FPL.

• **Omnibus Budget Reconciliation Act of 1990.** Medicaid eligibility required, to be phased in by September 2002, for children ages 6 through 8 in families earning up to 100 percent of FPL.

SOURCE: Mann et al., 2003.

of the income eligibility scale, take-up rates for persons newly eligible under the Medicaid expansions were relatively low (LoSasso and Buchmueller, 2002). The Omnibus Budget Reconciliation Act of 1990 mandated that eligibility for children through age 18 in families earning less than the federal poverty level (FPL) be phased in by September 2002, so that most U.S.-born children in this category are now eligible for public coverage.[13] Yet the latest Census Bureau data indicate that nearly a quarter of children in this income bracket remain uninsured; foreign-born children who are ineligible for Medicaid comprise a part but not all of this uninsured group (Ku and Blaney, 2000; IOM, 2001a; Fronstin, 2002).

The State Children's Health Insurance Program and Medicaid, 1997–2002

Finding: SCHIP has extended coverage among children to a significant degree and, to a much lesser extent to date, their parents.

Finding: The reduction in uninsurance achieved through SCHIP is jeopardized by the program's financing structure as a time-limited program of grants-in-aid rather than an individual entitlement.

Despite the Medicaid expansions of the late 1980s, nearly 15 percent of children under age 18 were uninsured in 1997 (Fronstin, 2000). Many of these children were ineligible for Medicaid because their families earned too much for them to qualify for Medicaid yet too little to afford private coverage. In addition, welfare reform in 1996 had led many low-income children and their parents to drop out of the Medicaid program because they did not realize that eligibility no longer depended on being a welfare recipient (Mann et al., 2003). In 1997, with a political consensus on the need for children to be insured, Congress enacted SCHIP as part of the Balanced Budget Act.[14]

SCHIP created a new option for states to use matching funds from a capped, ten-year grants-in-aid program providing roughly $40 billion to the states (fiscal years 1998 through 2007). Funds are unevenly allocated over the decade, with a "dip" in federal dollars scheduled for fiscal years 2003–2005 likely to result in program cutbacks (Dubay et al., 2002b). Most states quickly established their own SCHIP programs, structuring them as Medicaid expansions, as a new separate program, or as a combination of the two. As of February 2003, 19 states have

---

[13]Since 1996, welfare and immigration reform legislation has barred legal immigrants who arrive after August 1996 from eligibility for Medicaid, SCHIP, and other federal means-tested benefits programs for their first five years in the United States, except for the financing of emergency care, with exceptions made for specific categories of persons, including refugees (Rosenbaum, 2000). See discussion in the Committee's first report, *Coverage Matters* (IOM, 2001a).

[14]Title XXI of the Social Security Act.

BOX 3.4
How the State Children's Health Insurance Program (SCHIP) Differs from Medicaid Programs

Eligibility

Medicaid creates an entitlement for those who meet the eligibility criteria and SCHIP does not.[1] This fundamental distinction between the two programs means that states can reduce or eliminate their SCHIP programs at any time, jeopardizing progress in reducing uninsurance (Rosenbaum and Smith, 2001). States using the SCHIP approach can limit total enrollment even for those otherwise eligible for the program. While Medicaid recipients may also have access to private coverage, SCHIP enrollees must be eligible for no other type of public coverage and not be covered under a private health plan. While Medicaid eligibility focuses on pregnant women, infants, and younger children (children through age 18 are eligible if they live in families earning less than poverty), SCHIP makes age breaks in eligibility more uniform among the states and broadens eligibility up to twice the poverty level for all children (Ullman and Hill, 2001; Dubay et al., 2002a). Under Medicaid waivers, states have used SCHIP dollars that they are not using to cover eligible children to raise eligibility levels for low-income parents, either directly or by means of premium assistance to purchase employment-based coverage.[2]

Financing

Both programs are financed by federal matching grants to the states, but SCHIP provides a more generous federal match, although it is coupled with a cap on the total federal amount available to each state (Wooldridge et al., 2003). States have access to their annual allotment over a three-year period, with unspent funds being returned to the general pool of SCHIP dollars after that point and available to

SCHIP programs separate from Medicaid, 21 states have expanded Medicaid as their SCHIP program, and 16 states have combined a separate SCHIP with expanded Medicaid (CMS, 2003b).[15] See Box 3.4 for a description of SCHIP's key features.

The program was originally intended to reach 40 percent of children uninsured at the time, targeting children and families earning between 100 and 200 percent of poverty and allowing states to raise eligibility above 200 percent if their existing Medicaid program already covered children at twice poverty (Wooldridge et al., 2003). State SCHIP programs vary in their maximum income eligibility thresholds and in eligibility levels for children at different ages; on average, the proportion of children between 100 and 200 percent of poverty eligible for public coverage rose from 22 percent to 82 percent (LoSasso and Buchmueller, 2002).

---

[15]Note that the count includes the 50 states and the District of Columbia, plus 5 territories.

be allocated to states that have spent their entire allotment, unless restricted by federal rules. Unlike Medicaid, where premiums and copayments for children are prohibited, under SCHIP modest out-of-pocket expenditures are permitted within federal constraints (e.g., copayments, premiums, enrollment fees, deductibles) (Wooldridge et al., 2003).

Benefits

SCHIP programs created as part of an existing Medicaid program must offer Medicaid's comprehensive benefits package, while programs established separately are held to a lower standard, with federal law establishing the minimum benefits package required. However, most separate SCHIP programs include benefits more generous than the federally required minimums, with one-third of these programs offering the same benefits as Medicaid, and a national evaluation of SCHIP finds a consensus among respondents that SCHIP benefits packages generally meet the needs of most children enrolled (Weil and Hill, 2003; Wooldridge et al., 2003).

---

[1]Populations to whom states choose to extend Medicaid eligibility (so-called optional groups, rather than groups for whom the federal government mandates eligibility) may not be entitled to coverage, which may be restricted or withdrawn by the state at any time.

[2]Eight states have received waivers to expand eligibility to low-income parents and 7 have obtained waivers to use SCHIP funds for premium subsidies (Wooldridge et al., 2003). The new Health Insurance Flexibility and Accountability waivers, a revamped version of the Section 1115 waiver, are also being used by 4 states to expand eligibility to low-income parents using SCHIP, starting in January 2001 (Schneider, 2002; Wooldridge et al., 2003).

During 2002, an estimated 5.3 million children were enrolled in SCHIP at one time or another, about one-seventh as many as are enrolled in the Medicaid program (CMS, 2003a; Wooldridge et al., 2003).

In the process of actively engaging in outreach to build and maintain SCHIP enrollment, states have increased Medicaid enrollments (Dubay et al., 2002b; Wooldridge et al., 2003). A study of SCHIP at 12 urban sites across the country (representative and nonrandom sample) in 2000 and 2001 found that outreach strategies allowed states to overcome their initial difficulties in reaching enrollment targets and in some cases exceeding their goals for SCHIP, as well as raising Medicaid enrollments (Felland and Benoit, 2001; Mann, 2002). The states streamlined applications and application processes, used materials translated into languages other than English, and involved local community-based groups and organizations (e.g., health clinics, schools, hospitals, employers) in outreach campaigns tailored to reach groups with high uninsured rates (e.g., ethnic and racial minorities, immigrants) (Felland and Benoit, 2001). A follow-up study of enrollment between 1997 and 2001 observed a large increase during 2000–2001 and the biggest increases in coverage in areas with the highest uninsured rates for children (Cunningham et al., 2002).

As noted earlier, the design of SCHIP programs has reflected the concern that public coverage not substitute for existing employment-based health insurance (Lutzky and Hill, 2001). This concern is greater with SCHIP than with Medicaid because SCHIP has higher income eligibility levels, and extensions to parents and premium assistance for employment-based coverage are planned. Federal regulations require that states explicitly attempt to minimize substitution, for example, by requiring that enrollees be uninsured for a specified period of time before enrolling, as do two-thirds of the states (Alteras, 2001; Lutzky and Hill, 2001).

Because of differences in how substitution is defined and in analytic methods, no consensus exists about the extent of its impact. Some researchers conclude that the lack of affordable private coverage for families earning less than 150 percent of FPL makes substitution less of a concern. An interim evaluation of SCHIP in New York finds that only 4 to 6 percent of children enrolled in Child Health Plus had parents who reported dropping private coverage within the previous 6 months (Lutzky and Hill, 2001; Wooldridge et al., 2003). Alternatively, two recent studies of changes in coverage between 1997 and 2001 for children in families earning less than twice the poverty level report estimated levels of substitution comparable to early estimates under the Medicaid expansions of the late 1980s and early 1990s of between 18 and 50 percent (Cunningham et al., 2002; LoSasso and Buchmueller, 2002).

A national interim evaluation of SCHIP notes its successes in

- extending broad and affordable coverage,
- providing greater access to health care for the millions of children newly enrolled,
- securing ongoing federal financial support, and
- improving outreach and streamlining program administration compared with Medicaid (Woodridge et al., 2003).

Between 1997 and 2001, the proportion of uninsured children in families earning less than twice the poverty level declined nearly 4 percentage points, and there was an even larger drop for children between 100 and 200 percent of poverty (Cunningham et al., 2002). For children in families with income below the poverty line, however, the uninsured rate increased during the 1990s (Holahan et al., 2003a). For *all* children nationally between 1994 and 2000, there was a decline in public coverage, from 18.5 percent to 16.4 percent, and it was growth in employment-based coverage, reflecting economic prosperity and welfare reform, that lowered uninsured rates (Holahan et al., 2003a).

Despite outreach efforts and measures to simplify enrollment and reenrollment, SCHIP resembles the Medicaid expansions that preceded it in that only two-thirds of eligible children are enrolled (Dubay et al., 2002b). In 2002, there were 7.8 million uninsured children, and more than 4 million of these were eligible for but not enrolled in either Medicaid or SCHIP (Kenney et al., 2003).

Federal Regulation of Private (Employment-Based) Coverage

Finding: Federal initiatives to regulate portability and renewability of employment-based coverage have failed to reduce overall rates of uninsurance significantly because they have been too narrowly targeted and have not addressed the affordability of insurance premiums.

Because most Americans receive their health insurance through their employers or as dependents on another's employment-based policy, there has been much interest in reducing uninsurance by extending such coverage, through insurance market reforms or regulation of premiums, benefit packages, and eligibility. The federal government influences the degree of private coverage generally through its favorable tax treatment of premiums (the employer's contribution is tax exempt for both the employer and the employee). Although much of the authority to regulate insurance products is reserved to the states, the U.S. Department of Labor may regulate qualified employer benefit plans (including health insurance) under the Employee Retirement Income Security Act of 1974 (ERISA).

ERISA, administered by the U.S. Department of Labor, constrains the ability of states to regulate health care financing in the private sector. It was enacted as a reform of private-sector employer benefit plans, including health insurance (Butler, 2002). Large multistate employers supported preemption of state laws to avoid having to comply with often-conflicting state regulations (Fox and Schaefer, 1989). ERISA preempts the states from directly regulating health coverage plans offered by private employers ("ERISA plans"), although states may regulate the state-licensed commercial insurance products that some employers purchase on behalf of their workers.[16] The federal government, on the other hand, may regulate employer health plans under ERISA, imposing standards for services, benefits, and eligibility that can expand private coverage.

To date, federal regulation aimed at extending private coverage has functioned through three statutes whose intentions are to improve the portability and continuity of employment-based coverage. They include:

- the Consolidated Omnibus Budget Reconciliation Act of 1985 (COBRA), which guarantees that workers (and their covered spouses and dependents) enrolled in their employer's group health insurance be permitted to continue enrollment for up to 18 months after leaving their job (up to 36 months in special cases) (Meyer and Stepnick, 2002);
- the Health Insurance Portability and Accountability Act of 1996 (HIPAA), which guarantees that certain categories of workers, previously enrolled in qualified employment-based health insurance, be allowed to purchase coverage after they have exhausted their COBRA eligibility and restricts the imposition of

---

[16]The market of firms that insure their own health coverage risks is sizable; in 2003, nearly half of workers with health insurance were in partially or fully self-funded plans (Kaiser/HRET, 2003).

waiting periods for persons with preexisting conditions who switch health plans (Meyer and Stepnick, 2002); and

- the Trade Act of 2002 (TA), which provides a fully refundable, advanceable federal income tax credit for 65 percent of the cost of coverage for certain groups of workers displaced by international commerce and retirees and establishes new grants to the states to support administrative costs and state high-risk insurance pools (Dorn, 2003). This provision extends subsidized eligibility for a relatively small number of unemployed workers and their dependents, roughly 260,000 people (Dorn, 2003).

Because of federal preemption, state laws do not reach certain firms or types of coverage. But many states have similar or stronger regulations that preceded COBRA and HIPAA, such as guaranteed issue and renewal; COBRA-like provisions for small firms (employers with fewer than 20 workers are exempt from COBRA); restrictions on premiums; requirements that coverage be convertible to a nongroup policy; and limitations on insurers' use of preexisting conditions to deny or restrict coverage (Nichols and Blumberg, 1998; Gruber, 2001; GAO, 2002).

All three federal laws attempt to preserve coverage for unemployed workers and their families, particularly those unemployed temporarily. HIPAA also targets anyone changing from one employment-based plan to another. One recent study puts the number of unemployed at 8.3 million and those both unemployed and uninsured at 3.9 million, with an additional 1.5 million persons per month losing their jobs in 2003 (Etheredge and Dorn, 2003). Unemployed adults have an uninsured rate threefold higher than the uninsured rate for adults in the general population (Lambrew, 2001). About 58 percent of uninsured adults (point-in-time estimate of coverage status) report having changed or lost jobs in the previous year (Gruber, 2001).

Over the course of a year, workers earning less than twice the poverty level and their dependents are both more likely to be uninsured and more likely to lose what coverage they may have, whether private or public. They are more likely to experience changes in family structure that affect eligibility, more likely to change or lose jobs, less likely to be offered employment-based coverage when they are employed, and more likely to find COBRA unaffordable (Ku and Ross, 2002). Improving the level of coverage within this group would close a significant gap, as more than 80 percent of the uninsured are members of working families and nearly two-thirds are in families that earn less than 200 percent of FPL (IOM, 2001a). If all persons in households with incomes below twice the poverty line were able to keep their private coverage continuously over one year, there would be more than a 25 percent decrease in the number of uninsured adults and nearly a 40 percent decrease in the number of uninsured children (Ku and Ross, 2002). However, workers earning less than twice poverty are less likely to be eligible for COBRA than are workers in higher income brackets, reflecting the fact that many lower income employees do not obtain coverage through their employers or work for small firms (Doty and Schoen, 2001; Lambrew, 2001; Zuckerman et al., 2001).

There is little information with which to assess the success of COBRA and HIPAA in improving coverage levels among the unemployed. The lack of regulation to make premiums affordable to unemployed workers has seriously limited their impact (GAO, 2002; Meyer and Stepnick, 2002; Pollitz et al., 2000). The average premium bill under COBRA in 2002 is 102 percent of the full cost of employment-based coverage, or $288 per month for an individual and $771 monthly for family coverage (Kaiser/HRET, 2003). While three out of four workers are eligible for COBRA, only about 20 percent of those eligible take up enrollment under COBRA (Lambrew, 2001). A survey of unemployment benefits in six states finds that the monthly premium for coverage under COBRA would consume much of, and in some cases the entire, unemployment benefit (GAO, 2002). At the same time, in four of the six states, adults receiving unemployment benefits had too high an income to qualify for public insurance, although their dependent children might have been eligible (GAO, 2002). In 2000, more than 50 percent of the children of unemployed adults obtained coverage through Medicaid or SCHIP, compared with 9 percent of unemployed adults (Lambrew, 2001). It remains to be seen whether the 65 percent subsidy given to displaced workers under the TA's authority will make premiums affordable enough to increase insurance coverage among this group (Etheredge and Dorn, 2003).

STATE INITIATIVES TO EXTEND COVERAGE

In the 1990s, particularly in the years surrounding and following the failure of the Clinton Administration's proposed comprehensive health care reform, the states took leadership in efforts to reduce uninsurance within their boundaries (Oliver and Paul-Shaheen, 1997; Paul-Shaheen, 1998; Brown and Sparer, 2001; Holahan and Pohl, 2003). This section describes a key constraint on state options, the ERISA, and summarizes the experiences of five states—Hawaii, Massachusetts, Minnesota, Oregon, and Tennessee—that invested both funds and political capital during the 1980s and 1990s in programs that markedly extended public coverage and lowered their uninsured rates.[17] While many more states have established innovative coverage expansions in the 1980s and 1990s, the Committee has chosen to look briefly at five leading states whose efforts were both intended to and did have a dramatic impact and whose experiences provide a

---

[17]Lower uninsured rates are primarily influenced by a state's level of employment-based coverage and also reflect economic characteristics of the state or region (including the propensity of employers to offer coverage) and specific demographic and socioeconomic characteristics of their populations; limited evidence allows for the sorting out of these different influences on coverage status of state populations over time. See discussion in Appendix B of the Committee's fourth report, *A Shared Destiny* (IOM, 2003a).

comparison of different paths to reform.[18] These states have regulated private-sector coverage (employment-based coverage and individually purchased coverage in the small and nongroup markets) and revamped public coverage (both programs that receive federal matching funds and programs funded wholly by the state and localities).

Fiscal pressures on state governments and a growing unmet need for health services have catalyzed reform efforts to extend coverage. The need for states to stay within fixed budgets that cannot have deficits, to convince legislators to allocate new funds for public coverage, and to forestall the substitution of new public coverage for existing private coverage have stemmed the early ambitions of state programs to achieve universal coverage (Gold et al., 2001). In addition, state government's capacity to finance health care and coverage extensions tends to be weakest at times when demands for such support are likely to be highest, for example, during an economic recession (IOM, 2003a). Administrative barriers to enrollment, including those that discourage crowd out, protect a state's program from running out of money. However, these provisions can defeat the purpose of maximizing public coverage, for example, requiring that a child be uninsured for six months before becoming eligible for SCHIP. When states do lower administrative barriers to enrollment, the response can be positive and rapid. Box 3.5 illustrates one example, that of New York's Disaster Relief Medicaid program.

Starting in 2001, state efforts to extend coverage have been complicated by a period of financial stress on state budgets that has intensified with the subsequent economic downturn (Guyer, 2003; Jenny and Ferradino, 2003; McNichol, 2003). For some states, including the ones to be discussed, economic pressures have translated into cutbacks in Medicaid and other public coverage programs, with cuts in eligibility for parents and other low-income adults, the trimming of benefits, the addition of administrative procedures likely to slow or interrupt coverage, and greater cost-sharing (Fossett and Burke, 2003; Ross and Cox, 2003; Smith et al., 2003).[19] However, because state dollars spent on Medicaid and SCHIP bring in federal matching funds, states have made efforts to maintain their investment in public coverage (Howell et al., 2002; Boyd, 2003; Holahan et al., 2003d). State budget cuts to programs that receive matching funds result not only

---

[18]It should be noted that the existing limits to reform have motivated recent planning activities to guide new approaches that build on current programs. Starting in 1999, the federal Health Resources and Services Administration's State Planning Grant program has awarded three separate cycles of one-year grants to fund data gathering about state uninsured problems and planning for reform of health services organization, financing, and delivery to close the "gaps" left by existing public and private coverage in the state (Sacks et al., 2002).

[19]Recent passage of the Jobs and Growth Tax Relief Reconciliation Act of 2003 is expected to give states a new infusion of funds by temporarily raising the Federal Medical Assistance Percentage (FMAP), or matching rate for the Medicaid programs, lessening the likelihood of further program cuts (Ku, 2003).

BOX 3.5
Administrative Simplification:
New York's Disaster Relief Medicaid Program

When the twin towers of the World Trade Center collapsed on September 11, 2001, New York state lost its computer system for the Medicaid program. The dramatic economic and public health effects of the terrorist attacks on local residents, particularly low-income persons who lost their jobs as a result, were amplified by the threatened loss of public health insurance coverage.

Within weeks, the state of New York obtained a waiver from the federal government for a four-month emergency expansion of full Medicaid benefits called the Disaster Relief Medicaid program. Income eligibility levels were raised to the level planned for the state's Family Health Plus expansion (not yet implemented at the time of the attacks), assets tests were removed, and emphasis was placed on simplifying enrollment. Eligible persons could visit one of many outreach centers located around the city, be assisted in filling out the one-page application, and receive coverage immediately. Community-based groups and local philanthropies were engaged to publicize the program and participate in the enrollment process.

Disaster Relief Medicaid succeeded dramatically in raising public coverage levels locally. During the four-month period of enrollment, which ended on January 31, 2002, nearly 380,000 persons enrolled in Disaster Relief Medicaid, which is approximately eight times the number that would have been predicted to have enrolled during that time period in conventional Medicaid (Szalavitz, 2002). After the closing of the temporary program, the state began a more complicated process of reenrolling some Disaster Relief Medicaid recipients in the conventional program and dropping others from public coverage, returning to previous enrollment protocols for Medicaid that present many administrative barriers (Adcox, 2002).

Vigorous, community-based outreach and a streamlined, simplified approach to enrollment have been credited with Disaster Relief Medicaid's success in enrolling eligible persons where previously eligible persons encountered administrative and other barriers to enrollment (Russakoff, 2001). Latino and Chinese-speaking focus group participants in a recent study of the program cited their enthusiasm for the program, which they often learned about through word of mouth from family members, friends, and neighbors, and praised the relatively simple enrollment process, especially in contrast with their experiences and perceptions about the Medicaid program (Perry, 2002). Respondents noted their difficulties in obtaining needed care before enrolling in Disaster Relief Medicaid and reported increased utilization of services, particularly to obtain prescription drugs, preventive and screening services, and care for chronic conditions (Perry, 2002).

SOURCES: Russakoff, 2001; Adcox, 2002; Perry, 2002; Szalavitz, 2002; Doyle, 2003.

in lost coverage and access to care for formerly insured residents but also the loss of federal funds.

Despite budget pressures, over the past year reform advocates in a number of states, other than the five discussed below, have put together sweeping coverage extensions that have garnered broad legislative support (Associated Press, 2003; Orenstein and Fox, 2003). California, for example, has enacted a mandate, to be phased in over 4 years, that firms with 50 or more employees either offer coverage or support a state pool that provides coverage (a "pay or play" statute) (Freudenheim, 2003; Ingram et al., 2003; Rundle, 2003; Waldholz, 2003). If fully funded, the legislation is anticipated to cut the number of uninsured by one million persons. However, the law raises several ERISA issues and will likely be challenged in court. A second example, the state of Maine's recently enacted Dirigo Health plan, is intended to bring about universal coverage for the state's roughly 180,000 uninsured persons by the year 2009, relying on a mix of public and private coverage sources and financing by means of a premium tax levied on employers as well as federal Medicaid dollars (Associated Press, 2003; Carrier, 2003; Haskell, 2003).

The States and the Employment Retirement Income Security Act of 1974 (ERISA)

Finding: The federal Employee Retirement Income Security Act of 1974 (ERISA) constrains the ability of states to mandate employment-based coverage, one strategy to extend private coverage within their boundaries.

Because most Americans receive their health insurance through their employers or as dependents on another's employment-based policy, there has been much interest in extending private-sector coverage, through insurance market reforms or regulation of premiums, benefit packages, and eligibility. However, as discussed earlier in the chapter, ERISA effectively precludes states from trying to expand workplace coverage by directly regulating employers' health plans (Butler, 2002).

ERISA does permit states to regulate the insurance companies and the company products that the state licenses, but not self-insured employer plans (Butler, 2000). The statute has implications for the options for extending coverage, either publicly or privately. In the area of public financing, states can levy a tax on employers and insurers to finance a public coverage program (i.e., through a payroll, income, or other transaction tax), but the tax may not be imposed directly on an employer's health plan, and state assistance to help purchase employment-based coverage for low-waged workers must depend on voluntary participation by employers and cannot be mandated (Butler, 2000). Neither state nor federal benefits mandates (which also apply to self-insured plans exempt from state regulation under ERISA) appear to influence the decision of a firm to self-insure (Jensen and Morrisey, forthcoming). Although court rulings since the mid-1990s have given states more leeway to regulate in ways that may affect ERISA health plans, ERISA remains a significant influence.

In the shadow of ERISA, the states have largely been limited in their approaches to extending coverage to regulating their small-group and nongroup insurance markets and extending public coverage. The division of responsibilities between the private and public sectors and, within the public sector, among

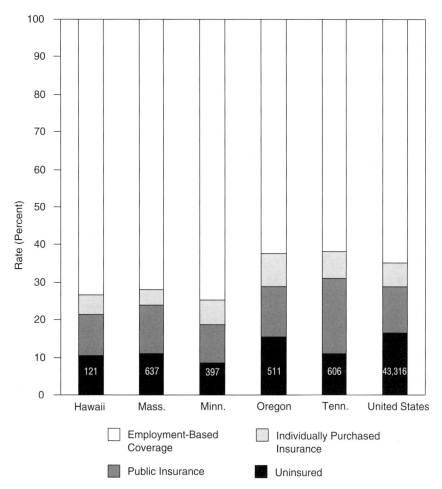

FIGURE 3.2 Coverage and uninsured rates and number of uninsured (in thousands) for population under age 65 in selected states and national averages, 2002.
NOTE: Coverage reported as military (i.e., Tricare, CHAMPVA) is counted as employment-based. Precise estimates do not add to 100 percent due to rounding and because respondents may report more than one source of coverage within a year.
SOURCE: U.S. Census Bureau, 2003d.

federal, state, and local jurisdictions, has made it difficult for states to fund public extensions for persons with incomes above the poverty level.[20] As a result, across the states discussed in this section, there is little variation in sources of coverage, other than the percentage of employment-based coverage; see Figure 3.2.

---

[20]See Gold et al. (2001) for a discussion of this "structural pluralism" and the inherent tensions and ambiguities that this pluralism engenders.

Five Leading States for Coverage Extensions

> **Finding:** At the state level, significant reduction of uninsurance is more likely with incrementalism that is integrated into a comprehensive reform strategy over time than it is with ad hoc or disjointed changes implemented without a plan to achieve universal coverage.

> **Finding:** Although some states have made significant progress in reducing uninsurance, even the states that have led major coverage reforms have large and persisting uninsured populations.

> **Finding:** Despite the use of federal Medicaid waivers to leverage the dollars spent by entirely state-funded public insurance programs, states do not have the fiscal resources to implement fully their existing public coverage programs. Reliance on income or sales taxes to raise revenues makes the funding base for public coverage programs unstable. States are further constrained from eliminating uninsurance within their boundaries by categorical limits on eligibility for federally supported public coverage programs.

In the sections that follow, the Committee highlights the differing approaches and experiences of five states that led reform in the 1990s. Since the mid-1980s, each of these states has taken advantage of Medicaid Section 1115 waivers to expand their programs beyond the mandatory populations and eligibility levels established by the federal government. Hawaii, Massachusetts, Minnesota, and Oregon folded in their own separate coverage programs for persons ineligible for Medicaid. It is important to note, however, that Section 1115 waivers do not bring new federal dollars into a state; all waivers are required to be cost neutral to the federal government. Following Hawaii's 1974 employer health coverage mandate, in the early 1990s Massachusetts, Minnesota, and Oregon each enacted and attempted to implement extensions of coverage geared toward universality, and Tennessee made its goal to dramatically increase public coverage. The experiences of each of these states points out the limits of reform without new federal funds. Despite the fact that these states started with broad employment-based coverage and public programs and have extended public coverage significantly, none has achieved universal coverage within their state. The progress they have made is now jeopardized by ongoing fiscal and economic difficulties facing states. Notwithstanding the recent passage of legislation in Maine that would move the state toward universal coverage, it is important to recognize that few states have taken on significant extensions of public coverage. Most states have higher uninsured rates than the states selected here for discussion and, thus, much further to go to achieve universal coverage.

Hawaii

Hawaii is home to nearly 1.2 million people of all ages, more than one-third of whom live in households earning less than 200 percent of FPL (KCMU, 2003d). The state has attempted to boost health insurance coverage through its employer mandate (the only one in the United States), called the Prepaid Health Care Act of 1974 (PHCA), and through public coverage. PHCA was enacted prior to ERISA and received an exemption from Congress in 1983 (The Hawaii Uninsured Project Leadership Group, 2002). PHCA requires most employers (with the exception of government) to offer coverage to employees working at least part-time (19.5 hours per week on a continuing basis) and makes a premium subsidy available to small firms (Law, 2000). Hawaii has addressed some of the coverage gaps left by PHCA through public coverage. A Medicaid Section 1115 waiver awarded in 1994 created the Health QUEST program, a capitated Medicaid managed care strategy that combines Medicaid, SCHIP, and state-only coverage programs.

While Hawaii's employer mandate has been interpreted as an important precedent for other states and a positive step toward universal coverage within the state, it is unclear how much implementation of PHCA has reduced uninsurance, compared to other factors including a relatively lower rate of increase in health care inflation, the particulars of the state's market for insurance (i.e., existence of modified community rating, small number of insurers), and health care utilization patterns (Neubauer, 1993; GAO, 1994). An 8 percent drop in the number of uninsured has been attributed to PHCA (about 8,000 newly insured persons), with socioeconomic and demographic characteristics such as the overrepresentation of Asian ethnic populations with higher-than-average coverage rates better explaining shifts in private coverage and the uninsured rate observed after enactment of the employer mandate (Dick, 1994).

Even with its unique exemption from ERISA, serious constraints on Hawaii's employer mandate have kept it from reaching its full potential. Criticisms of PHCA have focused on the state's lack of enforcement or oversight of employer compliance, the lack of a mandate that coverage be offered to a worker's dependents, and the fact that workers whose employers are excluded from the Act are most likely to be uninsured (e.g., temporary, contract, and self-employed workers) (Dick, 1994; Law, 2000); some of the difficulties with PHCA stem from the fact that the one-time exemption granted from ERISA did not permit the state to update or modernize its program once the exemption was granted, leading to administrative inefficiencies and in some ways a mismatch between subsequent needs and program capabilities. However, more than 90 percent of employers do offer their workers the option of purchasing a health insurance plan that includes dependents (The Hawaii Uninsured Project Leadership Group, 2002).

Because Hawaii's ERISA exemption has preserved PHCA basically as it was in 1974, the state's ability to modernize the program has been hindered and it has established other programs to cover the uninsured. Public coverage through

Health QUEST extends eligibility to pregnant women at 185 percent of the poverty line, children through 18 years at twice the poverty line, and other adults who earn less than poverty (The Hawaii Uninsured Project Leadership Group, 2002). Two other public programs extend coverage to those who would likely be uninsured otherwise: legal immigrant children ineligible for Medicaid and SCHIP and short-term coverage to persons earning less than 300 percent of poverty who no longer qualify for other public insurance (The Hawaii Uninsured Project Leadership Group, 2002). Funds to support the QUEST programs come from state general revenues, federal matching funds from Medicaid and SCHIP, and enrollee premiums.

The most recent Census Bureau estimates put Hawaii's uninsured rate for persons under age 65 at 11.4 percent (2002), lower than the national average though not the lowest in the nation, and about 121,000 people remain uninsured (U.S. Census Bureau, 2003d).[21] Of the state's uninsured, most are adults under age 65, although there are 24,000 uninsured children under age 18 (U.S. Census Bureau, 2003d). Three-quarters of the uninsured are in households earning less than twice the poverty line, for whom the uninsured rate is 22 percent (KCMU, 2003d).

Massachusetts

Nearly 6.3 million people of all ages live in Massachusetts, and almost a third live in households earning less than twice the poverty line (KCMU, 2003e). The state first moved toward universal coverage in the late 1980s and subsequently has significantly extended public coverage. Legislation passed in 1988 promised universal coverage, expanding current programs, filling in selected gaps and integrating certain aspects of the programs, and including an employer "pay or play" provision that was never implemented.[22] Voters came close to passing a second universal coverage referendum during 2000. In 1997, Massachusetts implemented a Section 1115 Medicaid waiver that broadened eligibility for existing public coverage programs, created two new programs, and merged the entirety into a unified MassHealth program (Bovbjerg and Ullman, 2002).

---

[21]The state's annual telephone Health Survey provides a much smaller estimate of 5.5 percent uninsured, or approximately 64,440 uninsured people, for the most recent year (2001) for which data are available (State of Hawaii, 2002; The Hawaii Uninsured Project Leadership Group, 2002). The state and Census Bureau estimates are not comparable, given differences in data collection, definitions of coverage status, and methods. For the states discussed in this section, the estimated uninsured rate is based on data from the Census Bureau's March Current Population Survey.

[22]The term "pay or play" typically refers to a requirement that employers either offer a health insurance plan to their workers and dependents or pay (often a payroll tax) into a public fund to support health insurance coverage for uninsured employees and families.

In the first two years of the waiver, there was a 14 percentage point increase in public coverage and greater than a 7 percentage point drop in the uninsured rate for low-income children; for low-income adults, there was an 8 percentage point increase in public coverage and an 11 percentage point drop in the uninsured rate (Bovbjerg and Ullman, 2002). Three years into the waiver, enrollment in public coverage had grown from about 700,000 to 926,000 (Bovbjerg and Ullman, 2002).

MassHealth consists of two programs that offer eligibility to the disabled and Medicare-eligible persons and four programs that extend coverage to the noninstitutionalized, nondisabled population (Bovbjerg and Ullman, 2002). These programs extend eligibility to

- pregnant women and infants in families earning up to twice the poverty level;
- children up to 150 percent of FPL, and parents up to 133 percent of FPL (Standard);
- unemployed low-income adults and their families earning up to four times the poverty level (Basic);
- children in families earning between 150 and 200 percent of poverty, adults earning up to 200 percent of poverty through an employer premium subsidy, and persons living with HIV (but not with active AIDS) earning less than 200 percent of poverty (Family Assistance); and
- emergency services (through MassHealth Limited) for low-income persons ineligible for other programs (e.g., undocumented immigrants) (Rosenbaum et al., 2002).

MassHealth is funded by state revenues and from federal matching funds from both Medicaid and SCHIP.

Massachusetts' uninsured rate of 11.3 percent (2002) is lower than the national average for the population under age 65. Nonetheless, there are approximately 637,000 uninsured under age 65 in the state (U.S. Census Bureau, 2003d). High levels of both employment-based and public coverage contribute to the relatively low uninsured rate (Bovbjerg and Ullman, 2002). Six percent of the state's children under age 18 are uninsured (approximately 88,000 uninsured children), and the rest of the uninsured are adults under age 65 (U.S. Census Bureau, 2003d).

Minnesota

A total of about 4.9 million people live in Minnesota, and 22 percent of them live in households that earn less than 200 percent of FPL (KCMU, 2003f). Minnesota has extended public coverage gradually, through a step-by-step or phased-in incremental approach of filling in private coverage gaps using the availability of federal matching funds through Medicaid to maximize the eligibility levels it can offer state residents (Chollet and Achman, 2003). In 1994, Minnesota inaugurated its own public coverage program, MinnesotaCare, intended to achieve universal coverage in ten years by expanding eligibility to all members of low- and moderate-income families ineligible for Medicaid (Gold et al., 2001). A year later, the state folded MinnesotaCare into a Section 1115 Medicaid waiver, together with the state's Medicaid program and other state-supported public coverage (Gold et al., 2001).

Minnesota's public coverage programs extend eligibility through a small group purchasing pool for county, town, and school district employees and their families; to childless adults earning less than 70 percent of FPL who are ineligible for Medicaid (e.g., noncitizen immigrants, persons in mental institutions) (General Assistance Medical Care); pregnant women and infants under two years at nearly three times the poverty level, families with children earning less than 275 percent of FPL, and childless adults earning less than 175 percent of FPL (Medical Assistance, MinnesotaCare); and a high-risk pool (Chollet and Achman, 2003). Because the state's public programs made children eligible well above 200 percent of FPL before the enactment of SCHIP and SCHIP funds can be used only to extend coverage to newly eligible populations, Minnesota's SCHIP program covers only a few hundred children (Chollet and Achman, 2003). Public coverage is financed with a mix of federal, state, county, and private dollars, including enrollee premiums and a tax on health care providers; about half of the state's spending is matched by federal dollars, for the most part Medicaid (Chollet and Achman, 2003). The state is at a relative disadvantage financially compared with other states because it cannot reap the full benefit of new federal funds for SCHIP that are matched at a higher rate than is Medicaid spending.

Changes in enrollment have reflected welfare reform and growth in earnings among the poor, for example, a dip in public programs (Medical Assistance and General Assistance Medical Care) after the delinking of welfare from Medicaid (Chollet and Achman, 2003). Over the decade from 1991 to 2001, both of these programs have declined somewhat in enrollment overall (although the numbers of enrollees outside of the welfare system grew), while there has been steady growth for MinnesotaCare (Chollet and Achman, 2003).

The state's low uninsured rate of 8.8 percent (2002) for the population under age 65 reflects high levels of both employment-based and public coverage (U.S. Census Bureau, 2003d). In 2000, public programs enrolled nearly all uninsured low-income persons under age 65 in the state (Chollet and Achman, 2003). Yet there are still an estimated 397,000 uninsured persons under age 65 (U.S. Census Bureau, 2003d). Most (325,000) are adults. About two-thirds of this uninsured population (including 91 percent of uninsured children) are believed to be eligible for but not enrolled in some type of coverage. If all eligible persons were enrolled, the state's uninsured rate, it is estimated, would stand at 2.7 percent (Chollet and Achman, 2003).

Oregon

There are approximately 3.4 million persons of all ages in Oregon, one-third of whom live in households earning less than twice the poverty line (KCMU, 2003g). Since the 1980s, health reformers have attempted to implement universal coverage in the state in coordinated phases. The most widely known of these reforms is the Oregon Health Plan, enacted in 1994, which expanded Medicaid (through a Section 1115 Medicaid waiver), imposed an employer mandate (never implemented because the state did not receive the exemption it sought from ERISA), provided a public subsidy for workers to purchase employment-based coverage, and created a state high-risk pool (Gold et al., 2001). The Medicaid expansion received national attention for its innovative benefits package (initially intended to be applicable to the employer mandate and other parts of the Oregon Health Plan), which ranked conditions by priority for coverage, given the budgetary constraints imposed by the Medicaid waiver obtained to implement the expansion (Conviser, n.d.; Skeels, 1994; Jacobs et al., 1999). Conditions for which treatment would be covered under the expansion have been ranked in order of priority (reflecting cost effectiveness, the number of people potentially affected, and other factors) and funding decisions made on the basis of the prioritized list. A series of working groups and meetings across the state engaged, and continue to engage in, public and legislative discussion about the scope of health insurance benefits.

Currently, the Oregon Health Plan extends Medicaid eligibility to pregnant women and children under age 12 with incomes up to 170 percent of FPL and other residents earning up to the poverty line (Gold et al., 2001). Through the Family Health Insurance Assistance Program, subsidized coverage is available for persons ineligible for Medicaid who earn up to 170 percent of FPL (Gold et al., 2001).

The Health Plan is financed by cost savings achieved through mandatory managed care participation by enrollees and state revenues including income taxes and a sales tax on cigarettes, a funding base vulnerable to change with the changing economic fortunes of the state. As a result, enrollment barriers have been raised to slow growth of the public expansion, through income and assets tests and premiums (Gold et al., 2001).

In 1993, before the Oregon Health Plan was implemented, the state's uninsured rate was 14.7 percent, or about 453,000 persons under age 65 (Gold et al., 2001). In the first year, there was an unanticipated groundswell of participation, with approximately 100,000 persons newly enrolled (the initial goal was to extend coverage to an additional 130,000 persons), of whom roughly 75,000 were new to public coverage (Leichter, 1999; Gold et al., 2001). Since the first year, growth in public coverage has been more modest, covering in total an estimated additional 130,000 low-income persons who would otherwise be uninsured (Leichter, 1999). Four years into the Health Plan, roughly two-thirds of the 1993 low-income uninsured population was enrolled (Gold et al., 2001).

Current coverage gaps include uninsured adults earning more than 100 percent of FPL, including those with incomes below 170 percent of FPL who, while eligible for the public subsidy, either may not be able to enroll because of fiscal limits on the coverage programs or may be unable to find affordable coverage (Gold et al., 2001). The state's uninsured rate of 16.5 percent (2002) for the population under age 65 is barely lower than the national average, and an estimated 511,000 persons under age 65 lack coverage (U.S. Census Bureau, 2003d). More than eleven percent of the state's children under age 18 are uninsured (roughly 95,000 uninsured children) (U.S. Census Bureau, 2003d).

Tennessee

Tennessee is home to about 5.6 million people of all ages, nearly 40 percent of whom live in households earning less than twice the poverty level (KCMU, 2003h). Although the state's insurance expansion was not expected to bring about universal coverage, it did broaden public coverage dramatically and significantly in 1994, through reform of its Medicaid program (Gold et al., 2001). A few years earlier, Congress had restricted the use of provider taxes to raise state matching funds for Medicaid, throwing Tennessee's publicly financed health care into fiscal crisis. State officials responded by obtaining a Section 1115 waiver that allowed the state to extend public coverage to greater numbers of uninsured persons and recapture federal Medicaid dollars that would no longer be available through the DSH program. The waiver created a new program, TennCare, that implemented mandatory managed care for all enrollees and doubled the number of enrollees within its first year.

TennCare extends eligibility for coverage to 400 percent of FPL. However, since January 1995, enrollment has been capped at 1.3 million persons because of limited public dollars to support further enrollment. Although TennCare is funded by federal, state, and local funds, including Medicaid DSH payments to hospitals and annual insurer assessments, support has been insufficient to cover all who are eligible to enroll and has also constrained provider reimbursements. One study estimates that, during TennCare's first five years, the federal and state governments spent about $700 million less than would have been predicted for the Medicaid program without the waiver. At the same time, TennCare's expansion of eligibility cost approximately $3.8 billion more (net new costs of $3.1 billion) from all payers than would have been predicted when anticipated changes in charity care, patients' cost sharing, and local government spending were considered (Conover and Davies, 2000).

At present, no new eligible persons may enroll unless they are members of groups required to be covered by Medicaid, dislocated workers, children in families earning less than 200 percent of FPL, and children in families earning between twice and four times the poverty limit who do not have access to employment-based coverage (Conover and Davies, 2000; Gold et al., 2001). In the year before TennCare (1993), Tennessee's uninsured rate was 13.2 percent (about 673,000 persons under age 65) (Gold et al., 2001). In the first year after TennCare began, the state's uninsured rate shrank by one-third to one-half, putting the state well below the national average uninsured rate. Four years into the program, nearly 400,000 persons have left the ranks of the uninsured and enrolled (Gold et al., 2001).

Currently about 12.0 percent (606,000 persons) of the state's residents under age 65 are uninsured (2002) (U.S. Census Bureau, 2003d). Most are adults, although nearly one in six are children under age 18 (U.S. Census Bureau, 2003d).

LOCAL INITIATIVES TO EXTEND COVERAGE

In many states across the country, counties are the providers of last resort for the underserved and uninsured (IOM, 2003a). Counties have responded to this charge in a variety of ways. The three counties reviewed in this section are among the few jurisdictions that have programs devoted explicitly to increasing the level of insurance coverage significantly and reducing uninsurance. Each takes a different approach, tailored to the characteristics of the local population, the resources available to deliver and pay for care that would otherwise go uncompensated or not be received at all, and local leadership. At each site, state or local conversion foundations, created as part of changes in the ownership status of health plans or hospitals, have contributed financing for coverage initiatives. From the following discussion of local extensions, the Committee draws the following observation.

> **Finding: Extensions of public or private coverage at the county level have focused on increasing coverage among targeted populations rather than the entire uninsured population locally. Despite the potential of local programs to address targeted gaps, the lack of a reliable funding source limits their scope and effectiveness.**

San Diego, CA

In 2001, there were nearly 365,000 uninsured children and adults under age 65 in San Diego County, or about 15.1 percent of the county's 2.4 million residents (Brown et al., 2002).[23] There is a sizable coverage gap among low-income workers. In 1997, two local organizations—the Sharp Health Plan (a nonprofit insurer) and the Alliance Healthcare Foundation (a conversion foundation)—created a small-scale demonstration program to reduce uninsured rates

---

[23]This is a point-in-time estimate (e.g., the survey respondent reported his or her coverage status at the time of participation in the survey). Analysts evaluating the county's uninsured problem developed a much higher estimate of the number of uninsured in the county, 537,000 persons, based on a three-year moving average of national Census data (the March Current Population Survey 1998–2000) that estimates uninsured status over a one-year period of time (the calendar year preceding the year of the survey) rather than a point-in-time estimate (Kronick, 2002). This higher estimate of the number of uninsured persons yields a higher county uninsured rate of 21.7 percent.

among low-income workers by offering employer premium assistance to small firms that do not offer employment-based coverage (Silow-Carroll et al., 2001). The program, abbreviated FOCUS (for Financially Obtainable Coverage for Uninsured San Diegans), targeted firms with 50 or fewer workers and formally began in April 1999.

Firms are eligible to participate if they have not offered coverage in the previous year, and they are given a two-year commitment of support (Silow-Carroll et al., 2000). Employees may enroll if they work full-time, earn up to 300 percent of FPL, and have been uninsured for the past year, with the requirement that all dependents be enrolled as well; however, dependents may also be eligible for public coverage (Silow-Carroll et al., 2000). Both employers and employees contribute to the premium, which is subsidized by private dollars from Sharp Health and two foundations (the California Endowment and the California Health Care Foundation) established when Blue Cross of California converted to for-profit ownership status (personal communication, Jeffrey Lazenby, Sharp Health Care, April 29, 2003). Providers are paid on a fee-for-service basis, and the benefit package is comparable to that of other local commercial benefits, with copayments but no deductibles (Silow-Carroll et al., 2001; personal communication, Jeffrey Lazenby, Sharp Health Care, April 29, 2003).

Although outreach has been an important part of FOCUS and the business community has offered much interest and support, enrollment has been limited by the availability of funding. To date, FOCUS has obtained roughly $3 million in private support (personal communication, Jeffrey Lazenby, Sharp Health Care, April 29, 2003). The target population initially identified was the approximately 49,000 adult workers employed by firms that did not offer coverage and the initial goal of FOCUS was to enroll 1,000 workers. As of mid-2000, nearly 2,000 workers and dependents were estimated to be enrolled, representing 232 businesses; participating employers are more likely than average to have uninsured owners who are also more likely to be foreign born and to have a very low-waged workforce (Kronick, 2002). An estimated 55,000 to 80,000 uninsured workers and dependents would be eligible to enroll if the program were expanded (personal communication, Jeffrey Lazenby, Sharp Health Care, April 29, 2003). At present, enrollment is closed to new firms but open to new employees and their dependents that join firms already participating in FOCUS.

Alameda County, CA

About 1.3 million people live in Alameda County, situated in the Bay Area and including the cities of Oakland, Berkeley, and Hayward. The county has an uninsured rate of about 8.4 percent, or roughly 109,000 uninsured under age 65 (Brown et al., 2002).[24] More than half of the uninsured adults are in the workforce,

---

[24]In 2000, the county supported its own survey of sources of coverage status over a 3-month

with 28 percent earning less than the poverty level and another 37 percent earning between 100 and 250 percent of FPL (Ponce et al., 2001). In 1996, the county health department began a collaboration with local providers, screening low-income people for Medi-Cal (the state's Medicaid program) for enrollment in a managed care plan (personal communication, Nina Maruyama, Alameda Alliance, May 29, 2003). The program, known as the Alameda Alliance for Health, has evolved into a private, nonprofit managed care health plan that receives a core of public funding and builds programming around its private-sector and foundation fundraising. Its goal has been to provide or coordinate seamless, continuous coverage for all members of families earning up to 300 percent of FPL who are county residents, considered as a unit rather than as individually eligible, regardless of eligibility for other public programs or immigration status (Ibarra, 2002). The Alliance's strategy has been to gather stakeholders and to participate in coalitions devoted to improving access to care.

Alliance coverage programs emphasize primary and preventive services while offering a comprehensive benefit package. Care is provided by a network of providers. Enrollees pay part of their premiums, with the Alliance supporting premiums that are not covered through public programs such as Medi-Cal or SCHIP. Copayments are tied to the type of service, with none for primary and preventive services to encourage utilization and a copay for emergency department visits to discourage nonurgent use. In addition, the Alliance takes a culturally sensitive approach to outreach among the county's diverse population, translating materials into a number of languages and working with community-based groups. More than half of the enrollees in its Family Care program are Spanish speaking and 19 percent speak Cantonese.

The Alliance offers subsidized coverage to all members of families earning no more than 300 percent of FPL (Medi-Cal, an SCHIP program called Healthy Families, and Family Care) and unsubsidized coverage (through the First Care program) for those with higher incomes (Ibarra, 2002). For Family Care, which has nearly 5,200 enrollees, family members may qualify under different programs, for example, Family Care program eligibility is extended to family members (parents, siblings) of those who qualify for Medi-Cal or Healthy Families. As of spring 2002, approximately 81,000 persons were enrolled through the Alliance, most of whom (68,000) received coverage through Medi-Cal. In addition, the Alliance Group Care program begun in 2002 offers subsidized coverage to full-time home supportive services workers (about half of whom were previously uninsured).

Financing comes from a combination of public and private sources. The

---

period, arriving at an estimate that roughly 16 percent of the county's adults, or 140,000 persons, were uninsured (Ponce et al., 2001). While this survey's estimated uninsured rate is about double the estimate given by a statewide survey that included a sample of county residents questioned about their coverage status over the course of a year, both surveys arrive at estimated numbers of uninsured persons that are surprisingly similar (Brown et al., 2002).

nonprofit's endowment is supported by grants from the California Endowment, the California Health Care Foundation, and tobacco settlement dollars from the county. Coverage programs have been added as new funding streams have become available, for example, through the federal SCHIP program (1998).

Hillsborough County, FL

In 2000, roughly 40,000 of the county's 1 million residents were uninsured and living below the poverty line (personal communication, Toni Beddingfield, Hillsborough Health Plan, April 30, 2003).[25] Like other Florida counties, Hillsborough (which includes the city of Tampa) serves as a provider or payer of last resort for the county's medically indigent population. In the early 1990s, rising health care costs, especially uncompensated care costs at the county public hospital's emergency department, motivated county officials to devise a health care plan for the portion of its uninsured population below the poverty line. The Hillsborough Health Plan is intended to promote the use of primary and preventive services, targeting low-income families and coordinating the provision of coverage with other public services in the county (personal communication, Toni Beddingfield, Hillsborough Health Plan, April 30, 2003).

Eligibility is restricted to persons earning no more than 100 percent of FPL; for persons earning up to 125 percent of FPL, catastrophic coverage is available with an income-based sliding scale premium (Hillsborough County, 2003). Enrollees obtain care on a fee-for-service basis through one of four networks of providers that have contracts with the county (personal communication, Toni Beddingfield, Hillsborough Health Plan, April 30, 2003). Since its inception, the plan has been supported by county revenues from property and a dedicated sales tax, as well as premiums for the catastrophic care plan (Hillsborough County, 2003).

The county made a concerted outreach effort through its neighborhood service centers and with assistance from local community-based groups, reaching an initial enrollment of 15,000 out of the 40,000 eligible (personal communication, Toni Beddingfield, Hillsborough Health Plan, April 30, 2003). In 2002, nearly 28,000 persons were enrolled in the Health Plan, divided between individual members (61 percent) and families (39 percent) (personal communication, Toni Beddingfield, Hillsborough Health Plan, April 30, 2003). In addition to extending coverage, the Health Plan has been estimated to have saved more than $11 million in hospital emergency department costs (personal communication, Toni Beddingfield, Hillsborough Health Plan, April 30, 2003). Like many other states and counties, however, Hillsborough has faced budget shortfalls over the past few years that have led County Commissioners to make difficult decisions. In

---

[25]A state-level survey in 2000 estimated the county's uninsured rate at 14 percent, with 117,000 uninsured persons under age 65 out of a general population of 839,000 (Lazarus et al., 2000).

2003, cost-saving measures have been geared toward decreasing enrollment (by requiring more frequent reenrollment).

SUMMARY

None of the reform campaigns or public initiatives discussed in this chapter has achieved universal health insurance coverage. Economic and demographic changes over time have influenced the level of private coverage (employment-based coverage), with larger public insurance programs such as Medicaid and SCHIP modestly lowering the proportion of uninsured persons by filling in some of the many gaps in coverage created by the employment-based system. As illustrated in Figure 3.1, however, given the absence of major federal reform targeting the general population since the mid-1960s, there has been little variation in the sources of coverage and in the uninsured rate over the past 25 years.

Those pursuing extended coverage in recent years have grappled with concerns and obstacles shared by reformers before them. During the era before Medicare and Medicaid, reformers sought health care financing arrangements that would apply universally (covering all members of society), be affordable to those seeking coverage, and be adequate in benefits to sustain health and well-being (making accessible the demonstrated and perceived advantages of medical care). The boom in private coverage between the mid-1930s and the 1960s, through Blue Cross and Blue Shield and independent plans initially, then by commercial insurers in the group market, made employment-based coverage the norm for most Americans.

Implementation of Medicare and Medicaid in the 1960s filled in some of the gaps left open by employment-based coverage, for persons aged 65 and over and for categories of the poor and medically indigent. The two programs, which today cover nearly a quarter of the U.S. population, grew to be much more expensive than initially anticipated. After the federal government became a major insurer and purchaser of health care, reform campaigns shifted their focus to controlling costs, stressing the need for insurance schemes to be affordable to society, administratively efficient, and transparent to political stakeholders. Over the decades, there has been moderate public sympathy for the general idea of universal coverage, yet no groundswell of public interest in a particular strategy to reach this goal (indeed, polls report a drop in support for universal coverage when couched in terms of specific provisions or financing requirements) (Marmor, 1973), and the spillover effects of a large uninsured population on persons other than the uninsured themselves have gone largely unacknowledged by the public (IOM, 2003a).

Even though most uninsured persons are members of families with at least one worker, government efforts to reduce uninsurance since Medicare and Medicaid continue to focus on public coverage to fill gaps. Since the mid-1980s, major federal initiatives to extend both public and private coverage have lowered uninsured rates among children and raised the numbers with public coverage, although the number of uninsured overall has continued to grow. Between 1984 and 1990,

Congress gradually expanded Medicaid eligibility for pregnant women, infants, and young children, delinking coverage from welfare eligibility. These Medicaid expansions were followed in 1997 by the creation of SCHIP grants-in-aid to the states. SCHIP appears to have reduced the number of uninsured children recently, but millions of children remain uncovered, more than half of whom are eligible (Broaddus and Ku, 2000; Dubay et al., 2002a,c; Kenney et al., 2003). Federal initiatives to extend employment-based coverage have targeted improved portability and continuity of coverage through the COBRA, HIPAA, and TA statutes, yet the lack of authority or resources under COBRA and HIPAA to make insurance premiums affordable has seriously limited their usefulness and impact.

With the exception of Tennessee, the states discussed in this chapter have relied on relatively high levels of employment-based coverage, plus generous public coverage for their low-income populations using Medicaid waivers and additional state funds to keep uninsured rates below the national average. Constraints on federal dollars, for example, due to the budget-neutrality requirement of Medicaid waivers, and the shortcomings of the federal matching formula (FMAP) to compensate adequately for the effects of economic recessions, contribute to the difficulties experienced by the states in extending coverage (Corrigan et al., 2003; IOM, 2003a). The federal ERISA also narrows state options to reform their private insurance markets, through which most of their residents obtain coverage. However, it is mainly the lack of sufficient or sufficiently stable public dollars that has checked broad access reforms, despite the willingness, albeit limited, of taxpayers in these states and others to tax themselves in order to raise funds to extend coverage, for example, through tobacco taxes (Marquis and Long, 1997; IOM, 2003a). Hawaii's inability to update provisions of its employer mandate to meet newer needs for coverage and failure to enforce the mandate contribute to an ongoing population of uninsured low-income workers, while limited resources have constrained public programs intended to fill coverage gaps. The breadth of Massachusetts' reforms is comprehensive, yet implementation of its "pay or play" law for employment-based coverage was delayed and eventually repealed due to waning political support, limiting the state's ability to boost private-sector coverage. Budget shortfalls have limited public coverage programs (MassHealth). In Minnesota, the uninsured rate is nearly the lowest in the nation, but gaps in coverage remain, jeopardizing its goal of universal coverage. The inability to obtain an ERISA exemption kept Oregon from using its innovative Medicaid expansion to broaden employment-based coverage in the state, and reliance on tax revenues has left the Oregon Health Plan underfunded. Finally, Tennessee's ambitious efforts to use existing Medicaid dollars and managed care contracting to markedly extend the program to its uninsured population with low and moderate incomes resulted in increased enrollment among the poorest segment of this group in the first year, followed by closed enrollments to all but those required under law to be covered. Localities, whose economic resources are more limited than those of the states (which can cross-subsidize among communities), may come close to filling a particular local gap in coverage but remain even more constrained than are the states by a lack of sustainable revenues for public coverage.

Despite gradual extensions of public programs at the federal, state, and local levels and isolated efforts around the country to move toward the goal of universal coverage, the lack of national political consensus has hindered a substantial reduction, if not elimination, of the problem of uninsurance in the United States. Laudable state- and county-level efforts to extend coverage have been constrained by a lack of resources. The circumscribed nature of these past and present initiatives suggests that attempts to provide universal coverage through state or local efforts without a substantial infusion of additional federal funds, and federal leadership, are unrealistic.

> **Conclusion: The persistence of uninsurance in the United States requires a national and coherent strategy aimed at covering the entire population. Federal leadership and federal dollars are necessary to eliminate uninsurance, although not necessarily federal administration or a uniform approach throughout the country. Universal health insurance coverage will only be achieved when the principle of universality is embodied in federal public policy.**

In the chapters that follow, the Committee builds on this base of knowledge about past and present efforts to reduce uninsurance to formulate its set of principles to guide a universal approach to insuring all Americans. These principles will be used to assess comprehensive models that describe "pure" or ideal approaches to universal coverage (for example, an employer mandate) in order to reach conclusions and recommendations about how the United States can definitely and successfully eliminate uninsurance among its population.

4

Principles to Guide the Extension of Coverage

The Committee believes the United States should not be bound by the limited successes and considerable difficulties encountered in past attempts to significantly extend health insurance coverage. The problems caused by uninsurance are too serious to be left unsolved. The overview of the Committee's previous reports and findings clearly shows that uninsured people have poorer health and die prematurely, compared with their insured counterparts. Having an uninsured family member can destabilize the whole family financially and threaten its well-being. Communities and their health care providers are threatened, too, when faced with large numbers of residents who do not have the financial means to pay for the care they use or need but go without. Also, the economic costs to society are large.

In Chapter 2 the Committee presents the key findings and evidence of its first five reports. That and Chapter 3, with its historical review of efforts to extend coverage and discussion of more recent federal and state efforts, provide the foundation for the principles in Chapter 4. The earlier chapters describe and analyze the evidence on uninsurance and previous attempts to reduce it. The principles in this chapter rely on that evidence without repeating it here.

Clearly, many more than 43 million people experience periods without coverage. There is constant movement into and out of insurance that results from the current collection of insurance mechanisms and their lack of coordination. Any solution that brings coverage to those without insurance cannot simply plug the gaps in the current "non-system." At a minimum, it must reform many aspects of current health finance and will, inevitably, touch on aspects of health care delivery as well. Optimally, reforms to increase coverage will improve both health insurance mechanisms and health care delivery. The first five reports of the Committee point to the need for a coordinated system of coverage mechanisms.

In this chapter, the Committee prescribes its vision for reform and a set of principles to guide efforts to expand coverage to those without health insurance that are derived from its work in this and its previous reports. Each principle relates to problems the Committee identified in the current non-system of financing care and outlines key aspects or criteria for our approach to health insurance in the future. Taken together, the principles provide a standard against which options to expand coverage should be measured.

The IOM standards require a conservative approach in assessing available evidence and using it as a basis for policy recommendations. Because this study has focused primarily on the effects of uninsurance, it does not have sufficient evidence to address all aspects of extending coverage and does not attempt to set specific criteria for all elements of financial access reform. For example, designing effective cost containment mechanisms is critical. Controlling costs would benefit efforts to expand coverage by making it more affordable. The Committee also recognizes the need for reform of the health care delivery system, as discussed in Chapter 1, but does not prescribe principles or criteria for all important changes.

The key goals of health care are to promote better health and well-being among individuals and to reduce the burden of disease of the populace. Based on the evidence reviewed and documented in previous reports, we posit a vision of health insurance for the country that is essential for achieving these goals.

VISION STATEMENT

The Committee on the Consequences of Uninsurance envisions an approach to health insurance coverage that will promote better overall health for individuals, families, communities, and the nation by providing financial access for everyone to necessary, appropriate, and effective health services.

Although insurance coverage is critical, it is not the only element of any plan to improve access to health care nationally. However, the independent and direct effect of health insurance coverage on access to health services has been documented in the Committee's previous reports. Insurance remains the key to opening the door to needed services.

The Committee on the Consequences of Uninsurance has formulated five principles to guide the creation of an insurance system that will help achieve its vision. These principles are intended to:

- consolidate all the Committee's evidence, findings, and conclusions into clear, simple statements;
- provide useful guidelines for policy makers and the public as they assess various proposals for extending health care coverage; and

- describe the characteristics of a better insurance system toward which we should aim.

The principles are based primarily on the Committee's first five reports; some are supported by additional research presented in this report. The statement of each principle below is followed by a brief description and rationale. The first principle is the most important and basic. Each principle is a necessary component for reform. The remaining principles are not ranked by priority. The Committee recognizes that any particular strategy to achieve universal coverage will entail choices to balance among these principles and choices to balance goals even within a single principle. The principles are purposely presented at a general level because the balancing of choices and the specific operational definitions of the principles will be created through the political process.

PRINCIPLES

1. Health care coverage should be universal.

Coverage for individuals is important. The health, social, and economic costs borne by the uninsured, others living in the same communities, and the nation as a result of widespread uninsurance lead the Committee to conclude that *everyone* should be covered by health insurance.

The Committee has documented the adverse impacts of being uninsured on the health and economic well-being of uninsured persons and their family members. Uninsured persons are less likely to get the timely and appropriate health care that they need. Compared with insured persons, the uninsured are sicker and die sooner.

The Committee finds that the adverse health and financial effects of uninsurance on individuals and families can affect others in the communities in which they live, and that the financial burden of uninsurance is spread broadly, if unequally, across all American taxpayers. The quantifiable economic losses associated with being uninsured are substantial.

"Universal" means "everyone." *Everyone* living in the United States should have health insurance. The Committee's analysis of the extensive body of literature concerning access to health services and health outcomes provides no evidence to support the notion that coverage should be limited based on citizenship or immigration status.

There are several reasons why it is advantageous to have universal coverage include *everyone* in the community. Newcomers (immigrants) are substantially more likely to be uninsured than are U.S.-born citizens (Hoffman and Wang, 2003). Because newcomer (immigrant) populations are often concentrated in particular communities and geographic areas, their uninsured status can have a more severe impact on health service providers there, particularly on emergency departments, than might be expected from national averaged data (Associated Press, 2001; Taylor, 2001; Gribbin, 2002; MGT of America, 2002). Also, communities with disproportionate levels of uninsurance have an added burden of disease and disability because uninsured people are likely to have poorer access to preventive care and worse health as a result. Vaccine-preventable and communicable conditions are of particular concern because they may affect many others regardless of insurance status if undetected and untreated (IOM, 2003a,c).

At the family level, U.S-born children of newcomer parents may be eligible for coverage, but if their parents are ineligible, the children as well as the parents are less likely to use health care (IOM, 2002b). At the individual level, many newcomers are working, productive, taxpaying members of their communities. It is only equitable that they also participate in the universal coverage strategy.

2.   Health care coverage should be continuous.

There should be no breaks in insurance coverage or periods without coverage because even healthy people can experience injuries or other unexpected health events that necessitate the use of health services. In addition, continuity of coverage promotes continuity of care, which improves quality (Weinick et al., 2000; Hargraves and Hadley, 2003). Having a regular provider of care, particularly for primary care and care of chronic conditions, is a generally recognized predictor of high-quality care and is also made more likely by continuous coverage. The Committee's first three reports describe how easy it is to lose insurance coverage, as well as the frequency and negative effects of discontinuities in coverage for individuals and families. About 80 million people were without health insurance for at least a month during a recent two-year period (Short, 2001). Uninsured spells can lead to poorer health, greater risk of premature death, and exposure to significant financial risk.

Employees and their families risk discontinuities because of a lack of effective portability of coverage when their job or work status or family relationships change. Much discontinuity in public coverage results from changes in personal circumstances as well as administrative difficulties related to enrollment and reenrollment. Some State Children's Health Insurance Program (SCHIP) requirements include having a prior period without coverage before becoming eligible to enroll. To achieve universal coverage, strategies to increase outreach and simplify enrollment and reenrollment will be necessary.

3.   Health care coverage should be affordable to individuals and families.

By "affordable," the Committee means that no one should be expected to make contributions to their health care coverage that are so costly that they cannot pay for the other basic necessities of life or afford to access health services. Because patient cost sharing at the point of service can deter use, no one should face a level of cost sharing so high that it would interfere with obtaining timely, necessary health services (Newhouse and The Insurance Experiment Group, 1993; IOM, 2002b). Criteria for affordability must be linked to income. For example, Congress determined that families eligible for SCHIP should not have to pay more than 5 percent of their income on medical costs, including premiums, copayments, and deductibles (KCMU, 2002b).

The Committee finds that the main reason most people are uninsured is that they perceive insurance to be unaffordable, regardless of whether the employer makes a contribution or insurance is available through the individual (nongroup) market. Uninsurance among families is strongly associated with relatively low income. Lower income families do not have much leeway in their family budgets to pay for insurance coverage and health services. Many experience hardships covering their food and housing costs, and low-wage workers are less likely to be offered health insurance on the job (IOM, 2001a, 2002b; Long, 2003). For example, without an employer's contribution, a family insurance policy comparable to the average employment-based coverage would require an expenditure of roughly 25 percent of pretax family income for a family at 200 percent of the federal poverty level (approximately $36,800 annually for a family of four).

Although some individuals and families with low incomes manage to purchase health insurance, the overwhelming majority would need a substantial employer contribution, government subsidy, or tax incentive to purchase private insurance or would need access to a nearly free public program.

As a matter of equity as well as affordability, people who are at risk of using or needing substantially more health care services than average should not have to bear the full burden of an extremely high out-of-pocket premium to cover those extra costs; the risks should be spread broadly. More than half the states have recognized this issue of equity and affordability and created high-risk pools as an alternative to *community rating*. The limited number of high-risk individuals in the pools and the level of premiums offered them in the individual insurance market indicate an affordability problem only partially ameliorated by the existing pools and more than 20 states lack even that mechanism (U.S. General Accounting Office, 1996; Achman and Chollet, 2001).

4. The health insurance strategy should be affordable and sustainable for society.

There is no analytically derivable figure of what is affordable to society. While people in Finland, for example, might be happy and healthy with total health spending at 6.6 percent of gross domestic product, it does not mean that the 14 percent that the United States spends is too high or that more would be unaffordable. Affordability will be determined through the political process and economic decisions made by individuals, families, and employers, depending on the coverage approach. The total costs of the benefit packages, subsidies, and administrative structures needed to support the health insurance approach should be affordable to society as a whole.

The sustainability of a given coverage strategy will depend, to a large extent, on the inflation rates for health care and health insurance and the ability to keep spending under control. During the past two years, high rates of increase in the cost of health insurance have contributed to employers shifting costs to employees,

employees dropping coverage that became too expensive, and states struggling to maintain enrollment, service, and payment levels in the face of rapidly increasing health budgets. A major reform to produce universal, continuous insurance coverage will need mechanisms to control inflation and utilization.

Sustainability also depends on a stable revenue source. The discussion of various federal and state expansions of coverage in Chapter 3 highlights the necessity of having sufficient and stable revenue to fund the expansion of coverage that can withstand economic downswings. This issue is a serious problem currently in states such as Massachusetts, Tennessee, and Oregon, not just historically. With increasing pressures on state budgets, many states are proposing, and some are implementing cutbacks in eligibility and benefits. The revenue issue is beyond this Committee's charge and further discussion of it is limited.

The Committee has reported previously the range and substantial amount of spending related to uninsurance, particularly by the public sector, and the dangers posed to the health care system by instability in public and private funding streams. Financing for the national health insurance strategy should be sustainable economically and politically in order to avoid the risk of coverage gaps and cutbacks in benefits.

Any new approach to health insurance should strive for cost effectiveness. To promote affordability and sustainability, the benefit package should encourage the use of cost-effective services and products through mechanisms such as variable patient cost-sharing and provider payment levels. Services proven ineffective should not be covered.

Because of the costliness of health care and because all members of society can expect to benefit from health insurance coverage, all persons should contribute affordable amounts through taxes, copayments, deductibles and premiums.

A new approach to health insurance should also strive for simplicity and administrative efficiency. In its previous reports, the Committee has found that the complexities of the current health insurance system make it difficult for people to use the system appropriately and obtain needed care. Some aspects of the current arrangements such as complex eligibility rules, underwriting, billing procedures, and regulatory requirements impede efficient administration. A new, simplified insurance strategy creates opportunities for efficiency and cost saving while maintaining the necessary administrative structure and control.

5.   Health insurance should enhance health and well-being by promoting access to high-quality care that is effective, efficient, safe, timely, patient-centered, and equitable.

The Committee endorses the recommendations of the Committee on Quality of Health Care in America that care and the health delivery system be designed to enhance the six aims for care mentioned above: care that is high-quality, effective, efficient, safe, timely, patient-centered, and equitable (Kohn et al., 1999; IOM, 2001b; Corrigan et al., 2003). To the extent that care is delivered more efficiently and effectively, the financing for it will become more affordable and sustainable for society. Payers, insurers, and those covered all have an interest in purchasing quality care, and the design of reforms in the insurance system should consider the impact on safety and quality of care. To the extent that reform of the insurance system affects health care delivery, it should promote those aims.

The best clinically relevant research evidence should play a role both in defining the features of benefit packages and in the daily delivery of care. Although definitive medical evidence and practice guidelines are not available for *all* services generally covered by insurance, they should be used when available.

The Committee has found that benefit packages that include preventive and screening services, outpatient prescription drugs, and specialty mental health treatment in addition to outpatient medical and hospital care are more likely to facilitate the receipt of appropriate care and better health than insurance that does not include these features (IOM, 2002a). The elements of the benefit packages should be updated as new clinical evidence becomes available.

Each of the five principles described represents an objective or goal for a more rational and effective health insurance system. Maximizing each of the principles concurrently may be difficult because of limited resources and political realities. For example, creating coverage with an adequate benefit package that is readily affordable to all individuals and families, yet affordable to society, will be difficult. Also, increasing the effectiveness of care will not necessarily improve its efficiency or make it more patient-centered. The degree to which the various goals are achieved will depend largely on the values placed on them by the public and the trade-offs made politically.

The Committee's role is not to determine the particular balance of these principles, endorse an existing proposal, or design a blueprint. The balance among principles should be determined through the political process. We present these principles to contribute to the public debate about insurance, enable informed choices about policy alternatives, and promote major reform. We note that some organizations concerned with uninsurance have developed principles for expanding coverage, many of which are similar to those of this Committee. Other organizations have gone beyond a statement of principles to design their own proposals to expand coverage.[1] The Committee recommends that the public and policy makers use the Committee's evidence-based principles to assess current insurance arrangements, evaluate options to extend health coverage, and, most importantly, overcome the present political stalemate to achieve coverage reform.

---

[1]The Healthcare Leadership Council, American Public Health Association, American College of Physicians–American Society of Internal Medicine, Association of Academic Health Centers, AARP, and Rekindling Reform Steering Group have each promulgated a set of principles to guide health insurance reform policies. The American Medical Association, American Nurses Association, and Service Employees International Union have each developed or endorsed specific proposals to achieve health insurance reforms, and other organizations and stakeholder groups such as the American Hospital Association, Catholic Hospital Association, and U.S. Chamber of Commerce endorse general strategies to extending health insurance coverage. See http://coveringtheuninsured.org/partners for further information on the policy positions of 17 organizations that support coverage extension.

The next chapter examines various prototypes of insurance systems that could achieve the Committee's vision of **health insurance that will promote better overall health for individuals, families, communities, and the nation by providing financial access for everyone to necessary, appropriate, and effective health services.** It will assess each model against the principles presented in this chapter.

5

Prototypes to Extend Coverage: Descriptions and Assessments

The problem of uninsurance has many potential solutions. Over the past decade, researchers, policy makers, advocacy organizations, special interest groups, and elected officials have all devoted considerable effort to developing proposals to ameliorate the situation. Proposals to extend coverage come from many different points along the political spectrum. Although few people openly oppose letting individuals have access to health care, opinions differ on how federal and state law, regulations, and public funds should be used and whether the goal of universal coverage justifies their use. Therefore, it is important to consider how successfully alternative solutions might fulfill the Committee's principles.

This chapter describes and examines four basic strategies to eliminate uninsurance. The purpose of this chapter is twofold:

• to highlight the range of options that have been proposed by focusing on four prototypical models that illustrate approaches under public discussion, and

• to demonstrate how the Committee's principles can be used to assess various options and thus promote a more informed public debate about solutions to the problem of uninsurance.

Each of the four prototypes satisfies the principles better than does the status quo. Each model does so through different mechanisms and realizes each principle to a different degree. The Committee does not recommend one approach over another. Rather, the analysis highlights aspects of each strategy that need further attention to correct a potential problem. Indeed, because the Committee chose to analyze very basic, simplified models in order to illustrate more clearly their inherent incentives, the prototypes lack some of the detailed refinements that have been proposed in the literature (Meyer and Wicks, 2001; Meyer and Wicks, 2002). If any particular approach is pursued, one will find many adjustments and corrective mechanisms available for developing a realistic and worthwhile strategy. The Committee cautions, however, that the pursuit of a "perfect strategy" could be an endless process and delay action unnecessarily. The Committee also notes that the four prototypes selected here do not include all possible approaches to achieving universal coverage and are meant to be illustrative of the variety of available mechanisms.

First, this chapter briefly examines selected design issues that must be addressed in the development of most proposals. The next section explains the Committee's rationale for the selection and development of these specific prototypes. The third section includes a brief description of each prototype. The fourth section assesses each prototype against the Committee's principles. The chapter concludes with a brief summary.

DESIGN ISSUES

Before addressing the specific models, this chapter identifies five issues or design choices to be made that affect many, if not all, of the prototypes. Aspects of the five issues are interrelated, but the issues will be discussed individually:

- voluntarism versus mandates and taxes,
- phasing in of target populations,
- substitution of new programs for current coverage and maintenance of effort,
- public and private responsibilities and functions for different levels of government, and
- risk selection and insurance pools.

This list is not exhaustive; the chapter does not attempt to cover all design issues that policy makers will encounter in crafting a reform proposal. These issues are raised explicitly now to acknowledge them and to identify implications of a particular design, not to recommend which choice should be made.

Voluntarism Versus Mandates and Taxes

The choice between policies that rely on voluntary action versus those that mandate a specific course of action is key. Most coverage extension proposals incorporate both voluntary and mandatory elements, but the balance or general level of compulsion varies significantly among strategies. Should certain players, such as employers, be required to provide insurance? Should anyone be forced to accept insurance? Can financial incentives alone induce voluntary universal take-up of an insurance option? If incentives can induce voluntary take-up, how much of an incentive would be necessary?

To cover the uninsured population, additional resources inevitably will be needed, almost certainly raised by taxes. The amount of money to be raised, saved through greater efficiencies or shifted from other uses, will affect the level, type, and sources of financing. These would likely vary among the models and would affect the political acceptability of any approach as well as its *equity*. New revenues are a necessary aspect of any universal coverage strategy. Based on estimates reviewed in *Hidden Costs, Value Lost*, we know that services that uninsured individuals use in a year cost approximately $99 billion (2001) and that additional health services for uninsured people would cost between $34 billion and $69 billion (in 2001 dollars) if they use the same amount and type of services as those who have coverage under the current system (IOM, 2003b). The program or budgetary cost of any fully implemented strategy would likely be somewhat more than the marginal economic cost of additional services, primarily due to shifts in the distribution of health care payments on behalf of both currently uninsured and currently insured people. These program costs would vary depending on the model and the richness of the benefit package implemented. Also, there would be costs related to additional utilization by some currently insured people if the defined benefit package for the uninsured were more generous than what they had and their benefits were raised to that level as a result.

Even if a successful extension of coverage were implemented, including effective utilization and cost controls, it is unlikely that a sufficient amount of the savings could be shifted to cover all the additional people because of likely resistance of existing stakeholders, discussed in Chapter 3. Also, the increased use of services by the previously uninsured would require some additional funds. Financing mechanisms, however, were not within the Committee's scope of research and will not be examined in detail in the discussion of these prototypes.

Equally important to the amount of new revenue is the issue of who bears the burden of providing this revenue—the broad social and economic impact as well as effects on individuals, families, and businesses. Significant redistribution of the benefits and burdens of coverage is virtually certain, and the distributional impacts will vary depending on the strategy implemented. In part these redistributive effects depend on whether revenue streams that currently support health services for the uninsured and insurance for the covered population are maintained or not. Such policy choices will be critical in the political debate.

The degree of compulsion (in addition to the newly required contributions) inherent in a proposal to extend coverage would affect both its political acceptability and its subsequent implementation and outcome, including how closely the model approaches universal coverage. Some mandates or constraints are unavoidable if universal coverage is to be achieved. A completely voluntary system is unlikely to achieve universal coverage, but the Committee acknowledges that trade-offs among the principles during the design of a coverage strategy could result in a reform that would not maximize the goal of universality. To assess the achievement of particular objectives, the Committee considers the balance of voluntary and mandatory action and its impact on various actors in the process.

Phasing In of Target Populations

Many of the recent extensions of coverage and current proposals target a specific population, such as workers losing their jobs as a result of international trade and retirees of certain firms that have failed to provide promised benefits (Trade Act of 2002, signed into law as P.L. 107–210), those leaving a job that offers benefits (Consolidated Omnibus Budget Reconciliation Act of 1985 [COBRA]), or children in families with low income (Medicaid and the State Children's Health Insurance Program [SCHIP]). The Committee defines its target population as all residents in the United States. Some proposals aspire to universal coverage but plan a phase-in over time, guided by priority populations to be covered. Defining the target population for an extension or a phasing-in strategy requires an early decision because it affects many other choices about mechanisms for extension. For example, if the first priority is to be the lower income, near-elderly population without coverage, lowering the age of eligibility for Medicare is an obvious mechanism.

The definition of a target population can require trade-offs between equity and program costs. For example, targeting the whole population within a specific low-income range for a new, publicly subsidized program or, alternatively, designing the program to attract only those who are currently uninsured within that income level would require different funding levels. If the former approach is taken, some people will undoubtedly drop their current private coverage. Everyone at a given income level will be treated equitably, but the cost of covering a given number of previously uninsured individuals will be greater than under the latter approach. This issue is also discussed in the next section.

Substitution of New Programs for Current Coverage and Maintenance of Effort

The issues of *substituting* subsidized or public coverage for existing, private insurance (*crowd-out*) and requiring employers or governments to maintain their current investments in health insurance (*maintenance of effort*) both relate to the preservation of funding streams that are currently being used for health coverage. Any new coverage program will alter, to some extent, current incentives for and behaviors of employers, employees, and various levels of government. The consideration of changed costs to various stakeholders is important in designing a new program because it is difficult both to change the flow of funds and to capture existing revenue flows through maintenance of effort provisions. The redistributive effects of any health insurance reform proposal will be greater if existing health care revenue is not captured or maintenance of effort not required.

The extent to which current financing streams are preserved or there are shifts in the sources of funding are key factors for evaluating reform proposals. To minimize the amount of new public funds that would be needed to cover the uninsured, some proposals for extension explicitly include mechanisms to discourage people from dropping private coverage they currently have in favor of enrolling in a new public program that presumably would be of lower cost to the individual. Other reform proposals explicitly intend to substitute the new program for existing ones. Although substitution of the new program may be desirable on its own merits, capturing the current funding streams reduces the need for new revenues.

Public and Private Responsibilities and Functions for Different Levels of Government

There are three basic questions concerning government responsibilities for major health insurance reform:

- How much responsibility should rest in the private sector and how much with government?
- Which levels of government (federal, state, or local) should be responsible for which specific operational functions?
- Which level(s) of government should take responsibility for financing, and who pays?

Answers to these questions would likely reflect a person's political assumptions and convictions, affecting both the scale of the whole proposal and whether it relies mainly on voluntary, private-sector efforts or public programs and policies.

Currently all three levels of government have responsibilities for providing coverage or care to the uninsured. The federal government acts as financier, providing a foundation of tax-based resources and setting minimum standards for eligibility and benefits for public coverage; the states share fiscal responsibility with the federal government, administering coverage programs (including making decisions about eligibility and benefit packages) and leading in innovative reforms; and localities directly support the delivery of health services (Holahan et al., 2003c; IOM, 2003a). Drawbacks of the present distribution of duties include inequitable variation in coverage from state to state, the relatively large fiscal burdens on the states for public coverage programs, and the fact that nearly one-sixth of the population is uninsured, with many of those persons eligible but not enrolled in public insurance (Weil and Hill, 2003).

The configuration of roles and responsibilities for health under the country's federal structure would likely change under any major reform proposal. One level of government or another might be more suited to specific functions, such as enrollment and its enforcement, regulation of insurance options, or selection of participating plans or providers. Responsibility for financing a reform proposal should relate to the fiscal capacity of each level of government. Areas of great need (with a high uninsured rate or large numbers of uninsured people) tend to have less ability to raise resources (Marquis and Long, 1997; IOM, 2003a). There could also be a mismatch of resources and need during weak economic periods, depending on what taxes are used. Financing considerations include decisions about the particular tax and source of revenue for the reform and which level(s) of government should collect the tax. How to collect the needed revenues, who should ultimately bear the burden, and how subsidies should be provided to those eligible for assistance are all design questions to be resolved politically (Wicks, 2003a).

How a reform strategy responds to the three questions posed at the beginning of this section will influence, to some extent, any redistribution of costs and payments. Some governments might benefit and others would not, likewise for tax payers. Also, to the extent the reform creates cost savings or at least reductions in the rate of growth of current health spending in order to fund the new coverage extension, there could be a significant redistribution of dollars. Given the natural inclination of all stakeholders to oppose reductions in their revenues and increases in their taxes, it is not realistic to expect that all current spending on uninsured people could be shifted into a new system. Nor is it likely that sufficiently strong mechanisms to control costs could be designed and imposed that would fully fund an extension to universal coverage. How much new revenue would be required for that extension of coverage would depend on the nature of the new strategy as well as on its ability to redistribute existing resources and contain utilization and costs.

Risk Selection and Insurance Pools

Insurance is based on risk sharing. A fundamental reality of health insurance is that the premiums of enrollees who turn out to be healthier than average subsidize the costs of care of those who turn out to be less healthy in any given year. Although a small percentage of the population (10 percent) generates a high percentage of total health costs (70 percent), just who will fall within that high-risk group cannot be predicted with any precision, and they are not necessarily the same people from year to year (Berk and Monheit, 2001).

Private insurance plans, with premiums based on the shared experience of a particular group of insured individuals, have a strong incentive to select the healthiest people they can attract so they can keep their costs (and premiums) low enough to attract more (low-cost) enrollees. Likewise, employers and individual policy holders have a similar incentive to participate in the healthiest and lowest cost *risk pools*.[1] These incentives are especially pronounced in the current small-group and individual insurance markets.

As a result of these incentives, older people, those in worse health, or those expected to have high health costs must often pay significantly higher premiums

---

[1]These insurance risk pools are distinct from purchasing pools, which permit small firms, associations, and individuals to join together to increase their purchasing power and potentially benefit from economies of scale.

for coverage. Some high-risk people are denied coverage and many cannot afford plans that are available. This is to be expected in a competitive insurance market and is necessary for insurance companies to be able to reimburse the higher level of bills generated by heavy users of services. Various regulatory and insurance mechanisms, such as *community rating, high-risk pools*, and *guaranteed issue*, have been used to help protect high-risk individuals from exceedingly high premiums. These approaches to spreading risk inevitably raise the premium for others in the pool, such as young, healthy men, or require implicit or explicit subsidies to maintain benefits. The size and heterogeneity of the risk pools, and whether the individual has the option to select a risk pool in any proposed reform, affects the long-term viability of the plan and the affordability of coverage for individuals and their families.

This discussion of design issues is far from exhaustive, but it indicates some of the choices to be considered in the preparation of a workable solution for extending coverage. Devising a strategy for increasing insurance coverage is technically complex. Technical issues often have political implications. Recognizing these preliminary and fundamental choices among reform options and engaging them early on should foster a more open political debate and ideally speed a political consensus on a particular strategy.

SELECTION OF PROTOTYPES

The Committee focuses primarily on proposals and strategies that eliminate uninsurance through *major, comprehensive health insurance reform*, rather than more limited proposals based on a discrete change to an existing program or a policy targeting a subset of the population. We recognize that the first prototype, which resembles many of the proposals currently under public discussion, is closer to an incremental approach than to comprehensive reform and would not achieve universal coverage, but it is included for the sake of completeness. Although reform around the margins may be helpful to specific subpopulations, it has proven inadequate in achieving the broader goal of universal coverage. Despite all the implemented extensions discussed in Chapter 3, the uninsured rate has remained high and is increasing.

We believe health insurance coverage for the entire population is of fundamental importance and value. Achieving it requires systemic reform. Even if small, piecemeal changes in insurance continue, they will not produce universal coverage in the foreseeable future. Universal coverage will require mandates, a significant change from current, voluntary arrangements. Major reform will take time to achieve, even recognizing that it is not necessary to design every fine detail prior to beginning. Modifications and refinements can be introduced during implementation. Garnering support for a comprehensive strategy and its implementation will also take time. Therefore, members of the public and policy makers should begin *now* to plan for major reform to achieve universal coverage.

Only a goal as important as achieving universal coverage that is equitable and efficient is sufficient to motivate and justify major systemic reforms. Even small changes can be costly, disruptive, and take time to implement (Marmor and Barer, 1997). The Committee did not presume to judge the political feasibility of various approaches. The historical record reviewed in Chapter 3, however, has convinced us that limited approaches, while perhaps more feasible to enact in the short term than major changes, are not necessarily better if they do not lead in the desired direction for future changes (Weil, 2001a). If the small changes do not lead to a more equitable and efficient insurance system in the long run, time and resources could be lost.

In the next section, the Committee examines four major insurance reform strategies and measures them against the recommended principles. Because these prototypes have not been implemented, there are no evaluations or hard data with which to assess the impact they might have. The Committee recognizes that federal policy makers and politicians face similar information gaps and uncertainties as they weigh alternative approaches.

The range of models draws on the breadth and variety of political viewpoints to create clear, coherent prototypes. They are arranged in order from the least disruptive strategy with the least change from the status quo to the prototype requiring the most change. Brief descriptions of the essential structure of each model are included. Some embellishing elements are included in the prototypes to describe a potentially workable model but are not necessarily inherent to a specific prototype. The four models were selected based on the following criteria:

• Aspects of the prototype are described in some detail in currently accessible literature.
• The prototypes represent general categories of approaches and techniques for extending coverage.
• They promise substantial increases in coverage, approaching universal.

The elements of each prototype were selected from commonly described strategies and seem inherent to the basic model. For example, although a single-payer model could have a more or less comprehensive benefit package or could have multiple benefit packages, we selected a single, comprehensive package for discussion purposes, because that is how the model is most often characterized. At a minimum, a benefit package in any of the models would include hospitalization and outpatient medical services.

Specifying a minimum benefit package for coverage of the *uninsured* would likely mean that people currently *underinsured* (with less than the specified minimum benefits) would need to be brought up to the defined benefit level to avoid inequities. Raising some currently *insured* people to the minimum benefit level would create additional costs. Improved health access and outcomes for the *underinsured* would also be anticipated.

In the assessment section that follows these descriptions, each of the

Committee's guiding principles will be discussed separately in relation to the basic incentives and effects of the models. The Committee does not attempt to estimate specific budgetary and private costs of the prototypes; much more detailed assumptions would be necessary to model the costs of each approach. The incremental economic costs of providing the uninsured with the kind and amount of health services used by similar people with either public or private coverage amount to between $34 and $69 billion a year in 2001 dollars. As previously mentioned, this estimate of incremental service expenditures does not assume any structural changes in the health system or reflect any particular model for extending coverage. Depending on the prototype and the scope and structure of the benefit package, the incidence and distribution of program costs would vary. Likewise, the health benefits of a particular prototype would vary depending on how fully covered the population would be and how comprehensive its benefit package.

In both the descriptions and assessments, the prototypes will be compared to the status quo. A summary table, describing the models, is included at the end of the descriptions (see Table 5.1) and a summary table of the Committee's assessment follows that discussion (Table 5.2). Each table includes a column for the status quo for ease of comparisons. The status quo is not presented separately in the discussions or intended as a prototype, merely as a point of reference. The current situation regarding health insurance coverage and finances is amply assessed in the Committee's previous five books and summarized in Chapter 2 of this report.

DESCRIPTION OF PROTOTYPES FOR EXTENDING COVERAGE

Prototype 1: Major Public Program Extension and New Tax Credit

This approach would make no fundamental changes in the current structure of private insurance. Some public programs would be merged and all expanded dramatically. A new federal *tax credit* (usable only for health insurance) would be provided to moderate-income individuals to enable them to purchase private coverage. The intent, ultimately, would be to make coverage available to everyone.[2]

Employers' Role: There would be no mandate on the employer. Firms would be free to offer or continue to provide coverage (or not) to employees and their families. Current federal tax incentives for employers and their workers would remain.

---

[2]Aspects of this prototype have been discussed in the following articles: Loprest and Uccello (1997); Davis et al. (2000); Hacker (2001); Short et al. (2001); Johnson et al. (2002); Morone (2002); and Davis and Schoen (2003). References for tax credits are mentioned under Prototype 3.

Individuals' Role: Workers and their dependents would be free to acquire insurance from their employer, if offered, or from the individual market (without the tax incentive), but they would not be required to obtain coverage. Individuals with family income above the eligibility limit of the public program, but below the level at which private insurance becomes affordable, would receive a subsidy in the form of a federal tax credit, if they chose to purchase insurance. The tax credit would be both refundable, meaning those with income sufficiently low that they would owe no tax would receive the credit as a refund, and advanceable, so that people would receive the credit upon purchase of a policy rather than after the end of the tax year. The tax credit would be used to purchase acceptable employment-based or other group coverage or a policy from the individual (nongroup) market. The tax credit would be sufficiently large for those with incomes just above the eligibility limit for public coverage and would phase out to zero at the point where family income would make coverage affordable without assistance.

Public Programs: Medicaid (except for the long-term care benefit) and SCHIP would be merged into a new single program run and funded jointly by the federal government and the states. It would offer comprehensive benefits, similar to those currently offered, with minimal cost sharing. Individuals up to a certain income level for a given family size would be eligible without regard to family structure or employment status. The eligibility age for Medicare would be extended downward so that individuals could enroll at age 55 with the payment of a special premium.

Federal and State Insurance Regulation: The federal government would establish an actuarial value or a package of services commensurate with the amount of the tax credit. It would be the insurers' responsibility to sell actuarial equivalents or plans superior to the federally defined package. The state would certify whether specific policies met the federal standards. The benefits would likely be less than comprehensive, limited by the size of the tax credit. However, the credit could be used for other, more comprehensive policies that would be available to purchasers paying additional premiums. Except for insurance offered for purchase through a tax credit, there would be no required change in the benefit structures of insurance offered or in public regulation of it. Hence, *affinity groups* and other risk-pooling mechanisms would be available in states where they are currently permitted.

Design Alternative: The new tax credit could be made available to low-income families, giving them the option of enrolling in public coverage or purchasing private coverage on their own with the subsidy. This model could also be combined with a subsidy for employers of low-wage workers in the form of tax credits, based on payroll or other business taxes, to encourage them to offer coverage to their employees.

Prototype 2: Employer Mandate, Premium Subsidy, and Individual Mandate

The current amalgam of employment-based insurance and public coverage would form the foundation of this model. The main change from the current system would be mandates requiring all employers to provide coverage for their workers and requiring all workers to take that coverage. Because employers of low-wage workers are less likely to offer coverage and low-wage workers are less likely to take up offered coverage (Kaiser/HRET, 2003), this prototype includes a premium subsidy for employers of low-wage workers to keep the insurance offer affordable to their workers. Subsidized enrollment in private coverage through a *purchasing pool* or enrollment in a combined Medicaid/SCHIP public program would be required of those who do not obtain coverage elsewhere.[3]

Employer Mandate and Subsidy: Employers would be required to provide coverage and finance a portion of health benefits for workers and their families, including, at a minimum, a federally defined benefit package. The package would be defined either by specific services or given an actuarial value, likely following the scope of current employment-based coverage, which is generally comprehensive. Firms would have to finance a substantial portion of the premium expense for all employees who worked more than some predetermined amount of time per week and their dependents. A protocol would be established to assign coverage responsibility to one employer for employees in families with more than one worker. Small employers and the self-employed would also need to meet these requirements and offer coverage. Because many small employers have low-wage workers, they would be eligible for a premium subsidy. The current tax provision that excludes the employer's share of the insurance premium from the employee's taxable income would remain, as would the employers' tax deduction and the deduction for the self-employed.

An additional federal premium subsidy would be provided to employers, including those self-employed, based on the firm's average wages in order to make coverage (premium and other cost sharing) more affordable for even low-wage workers. States would assist in the formation of large purchasing pools, particularly for small employers, the self-employed, other employers not already providing coverage, and those individuals not able to obtain health insurance through their employer.

---

[3]Various aspects of this model are presented in the following articles: Krueger and Reinhardt (1994); McArdle (1994); Steuerle (1994); U.S. Government Accounting Office (2000); Curtis et al. (2001); Feder et al. (2001); Wicks (2003b).

Individual Mandate and Subsidy: Individuals eligible for coverage at work would be required to enroll themselves and their families unless they showed evidence that they had obtained coverage from another source. The premium subsidy to the employer would be designed to make the offered coverage affordable for the employee. People who did not obtain coverage elsewhere would be required to enroll in a public program or purchase coverage from a large purchasing pool. Income-related subsidies would be made available to these individuals and their families not receiving employment-based insurance.

Public Programs: Medicaid, except for the long-term care benefit, and SCHIP would be combined into one public program (federal, state, or jointly run) that offered a basic benefit package for all those not in the workforce or insured through a working family member. There would be in effect a larger subsidy in the form of more comprehensive Medicaid-style benefits and more limited cost sharing for those with lower incomes. The public program could have a mechanism to pick up temporarily unemployed workers and those workers on a part-time schedule, including those self-employed and working only part-time, who did not reach the minimum hours for employment coverage. Workers who lost their jobs or were otherwise temporarily unemployed would enroll in the public program unless they preferred purchasing private coverage through a large pool. Lack of employment-based insurance or nonparticipation in the workforce (for the hours required for coverage) would be the only requirements for eligibility. The public program would require premiums from those of moderate income or higher and some cost sharing from all at the point of service. There would also be a public (federal and state) role in enforcing the mandates, regulating the insurance options, and organizing the large purchasing pools. This prototype would not change Medicare.

Design Alternative: The employers' mandate could be converted to a "pay or play" requirement. Employers that preferred not to provide coverage might choose to pay a payroll tax instead. Their employees would then be required to obtain coverage through the public program supported in part by that payroll tax.

Prototype 3: Individual Mandate and Tax Credit

Individuals would be responsible for providing health insurance for themselves and their families under this prototype. They would receive a subsidy in the form of an income-related, refundable, and advanceable federal tax credit for purchasing health insurance and they would be able to choose from a range of plans.[4]

---

[4]Tax credits have been discussed widely, including the following articles: Pauly and Herring (2001); Blumberg (2001); Butler (2001); Gabel et al. (2002); Hadley and Reschovsky (2002); Curtis and Neuschler (2002); Pauly and Nichols (2002).

Individual Mandate: Individuals would be required to purchase a policy with at least a basic benefit package that met federal standards to cover themselves and their dependents. Individuals would be allowed to purchase insurance from a variety of sources: through their employer, if offered; on their own in the individual market; or through a group purchasing vehicle created and maintained by the states or other organizations. There would be a mechanism, perhaps linked to federal income tax returns, to certify that the individual and dependents had purchased an acceptable policy. This insurance approach would eliminate the exemption of the premium for employment-based coverage from taxable income.

Individual Subsidy: The subsidy would go to the individual or family, based on income and family size. It would be progressive, phasing out above some reasonable income level. The subsidy would be made in the form of a refundable, advanceable federal income tax credit that could be used only for purchase of accredited insurance coverage. The insurance could be purchased through an employer or other group or a policy on the individual, nongroup market.

Federal and State Insurance Regulation: A federal agency, probably the Internal Revenue Service, which is separate and distinct from the regulation of health insurance, would administer the tax credit much as in Prototype 1. The regulation of insurance would remain at the state level, and each state would require the guaranteed issue (i.e., without regard to health status) of at least one basic and one comprehensive plan and at least one *medical savings account* along with a catastrophic coverage package. The state would also certify which plans meet federal standards. Groups of all kinds—employers, state sponsored, unions, and private associations—would be allowed to offer insurance and guidance in the purchase of acceptable plans. States would have the option to create large purchasing pools to assist small employers and individual purchasers, based on federal standards supporting the viability of purchasing pools. Employers could continue to offer coverage and could subsidize the premium. Although their premium contributions would remain a business expense for the employer, any premium contribution from the employer would be treated as taxable income to the employee.

Public Programs: The federal government would design and operate a program to provide the income-related tax credit to assist individuals in the purchase of insurance. Medicaid (except for the long-term care benefit) and SCHIP would be eliminated. Present enrollees of those programs and other low-income individuals would receive a tax credit of a larger size, designed to enable them to select and purchase a more comprehensive benefit package than that mandated for all, including reduced copayments and medical support services such as those covered by Medicaid. The more comprehensive benefit package would cover the broad range of services currently provided in the Medicaid program. Medicare as currently constituted would remain intact in this prototype.

Design Alternative: There would be an expanded state role to regulate the small-group and individual (nongroup) insurance market based on federal standards that would define a level of uniformity across states. For example, in addition to guaranteed issue, the state could require that all plans limit *preexisting condition exclusions*, adjust risk pools, or offer *reinsurance* mechanisms to keep premiums within certain affordable limits, and provide the option for people to use their tax credit to purchase state employee benefits.[5]

Prototype 4: Single Payer

A single payer system would mandate coverage for every individual, provide comprehensive benefits, be administered at the federal level of government, and be funded by federal taxes.[6]

Payer: The federal government would operate a single payer system centrally and make all payments to providers of services. A federal agency would administer the program, setting policy and standards for participation by providers and provider systems. The agency could contract with private organizations to review claims and process payments, much as Medicare now does. This model would require minimal determinations of eligibility and enrollment, and would standardize billing functions.

Benefit Package: The single benefit package would include all services generally considered necessary. The services included in the benefit package would be determined by the federal administrative agency, based on clinical evidence. There might be a role for *supplemental coverage*, such as Medigap or policies to cover nonessential services and amenities.[7] The definition of the single payer model requires comprehensive benefits so that it can achieve various efficiencies through control over most of the spending. Minimal copayments would be due at the point of service. No premiums would be required. *Integrated delivery systems* could offer delivery system alternatives to standard *fee-for-service* care (nonintegrated care delivery arrangements).[8]

---

[5]Through reinsurance the state would, in effect, accept part of the risk of losses underwritten by private insurers in the state, enabling them to limit their premiums for higher risk individuals.

[6]Various aspects of single payer models have been discussed broadly, including in the following articles: Beauchamp and Rouse (1990); Sheils et al. (1992); Gruber and Hanratty (1995); Norato (1997); Chollet et al. (2002); Himmelstein and Woolhandler (2003).

[7]Supplemental coverage in the Medicare program (Medigap) is private health insurance designed to cover expenses not paid by Medicare.

[8]Integrated delivery systems usually are interconnected, and cooperating organizations include hospitals and physician groups which provide or arrange to provide a coordinated continuum of services to a defined population and may be held both clinically and fiscally accountable for the health outcomes of the population.

Global Budget: A budget set to cover anticipated use by the whole population would control aggregate health care spending for the country. It would be necessary to design payment mechanisms appropriate for both the integrated delivery systems and fee-for-service providers, taking into account possible differences in levels of health status among the respective populations served. Payment rates would be negotiated between the federal agency and providers of services, drugs, supplies, and equipment, creating a system of administered prices for medical care.

Public Programs: With everyone enrolled in a single payer system with virtually no financial barriers to care, the need for Medicaid and SCHIP for lower income individuals and families would be obviated. Medicaid currently covers some non-medical health and social services, such as case management during pregnancy and transportation to care, to facilitate appropriate use of medical services by very low-income people. Those services would continue to be offered by the state through a different agency that would use another funding source. Thus, Medicaid and SCHIP would be eliminated, except for a residual long-term care benefit. With a single payer program of comprehensive public coverage for everyone up to age 65, it would be logical to incorporate the current Medicare program for the elderly into the single payer system so that people would not be forced, at age 65, into the currently more limited Medicare program. If Medicare were incorporated into the single payer program, this prototype would cover the whole population, including those over age 65.

Design Alternative: A single payer system could impose significant cost sharing at the point of service rather than the minimal amounts of the original model. This design alternative would likely generate greater demand for supplemental, wrap-around health insurance to cover those copayments and additional desired services beyond the comprehensive package. This demand could stimulate a larger market for Medigap-like supplemental coverage if people chose to insure against the risk of substantial cost sharing. Individuals and families of lower income would receive a publicly provided supplemental insurance package with no premium so their cost sharing would not increase.

See Table 5.1 for a summary description of each of the prototypes.

ASSESSMENT OF PROTOTYPES FOR EXTENDING COVERAGE

The following assessments address various features of each prototype in terms of the five basic principles for reform.[9]

---

[9]The principles are fully described in Chapter 4.

Health Care Coverage Should Be Universal

Prototype 1: Major Public Program Extension and New Tax Credit

This health insurance strategy would not achieve universal or near universal coverage because there are no mandates on employers to offer coverage or on individuals to obtain it. Based strictly on voluntary action, some people would choose not to purchase insurance or decline to participate in a public program. Such incremental approaches in the past have failed to achieve universality. Many of the barriers that now leave millions of eligible people uninsured would prevail. Nonetheless, the higher income levels covered by the public program, the extended eligibility for Medicare, and the larger tax incentives are likely to result in substantially greater numbers of people covered.

Prototype 2: Employer Mandate, Premium Subsidy, and Individual Mandate

Coverage under this prototype would be close to universal because all employers would be required to offer affordable insurance and individuals would be required to have some form of coverage: through employment-based insurance (their own or a family member's), through a state-operated large purchasing pool, or through the public program. An enforcement mechanism, perhaps through current business tax filings, would be necessary to ensure that all employers complied and offered coverage. To ensure that all individuals obtained coverage, certification might be made on individual and family federal income tax returns. Universality of coverage would depend on voluntary compliance and the effectiveness of the mandates' enforcement.

Prototype 3: Individual Mandate and Tax Credit

Coverage would be nearly universal. Because everyone would be required to obtain coverage, the effectiveness of the mandate would depend on voluntary compliance and enforcement. Consumer education and an adequately sized tax credit relative to the cost of available, certified policies would help increase compliance and minimize enforcement efforts.

Prototype 4: Single Payer

This prototype is designed to cover the entire population (or all those under age 65). Coverage would be universal because this strategy would be mandatory. It would require little enrollment data, no eligibility determinations, nor any reenrollment procedures. No premium would be charged to enrollees so a financial deterrent to enrollment would be avoided. If individuals failed to enroll initially, they would automatically be enrolled when they first sought service, making enforcement of the individual mandate relatively simple.

TABLE 5.1 Summary Description of Prototypes

	Status Quo	Prototype 1 Major Public Program Extension and New Tax Credit
Subsidies	Favorable federal tax treatment for employment-based coverage	Current federal tax treatment for employment-based coverage; federal tax credit for moderate-income people to purchase employer's plan or individual insurance
Mandates	None	None
Government Roles	Congress sets mandatory and optional eligibility for public coverage and regulates employment-based coverage; federal agencies define basic Medicaid, SCHIP benefits packages, and finance jointly with states; joint regulation of employment-based coverage; states administer public coverage (Medicaid, SCHIP) and define optional eligibility, offer state-funded coverage programs, regulate small group and nongroup insurance markets	Federal agency implements tax credit
Public Programs	Federal and state funding of public coverage for seniors, disabled, and categories of the poor: Medicare, Medicaid, SCHIP, and programs at the state and local levels	Medicaid and SCHIP combined and expanded, comprehensive benefits, minimal cost sharing; Medicare expanded to 55-year-olds
Private Health Insurance	Two-thirds of all insurance purchased through workplace, small proportion purchased in small group and nongroup markets	Current private group and nongroup insurance markets

Prototype 2	Prototype 3	Prototype 4
Employer Mandate, Premium Subsidy, and Individual Mandate	Individual Mandate and Tax Credit	Single Payer
Federal premium subsidy to employers with low-wage workforce, passed on to employee in affordable health benefit; current federal tax treatment for employment-based coverage	Individual/family federal tax credit based on family income and size; refundable, advanceable	Federal funding of program with minimal cost sharing
Employers must offer qualified insurance to workers; individuals must obtain coverage from employer, private market, or public program	Individuals must purchase qualified coverage	Individuals must enroll
Public agency(ies) provides subsidy for employers; defines basic benefit package; enforces mandates; organizes purchasing pools	Federal agency defines basic benefit package and certifies acceptable plans; another federal agency administers and enforces tax credits; state operates purchasing pools	Federal agency administers program, global budget, and payments through contractors and private health plans
Medicaid and SCHIP combined for all without employment-based coverage; income-related premiums; no change to Medicare	Medicaid and SCHIP eliminated; no change to Medicare	Medicaid and SCHIP eliminated; Medicare possibly integrated
Offered through purchasing pools	All insurance private, purchased individually, or through groups or state purchasing pools	Supplemental policies optional for noncovered services and amenities

Continued

TABLE 5.1 Continued

	Status Quo	Prototype 1 Major Public Program Extension and New Tax Credit
Benefit Package	Mixed private benefits; mandatory basic packages for Medicare and Medicaid programs	Comprehensive public program; private benefits mixed as currently
Design Alternative	Not applicable	Tax credit for lower income people with option to purchase public or private coverage

Health Care Coverage Should Be Continuous

Prototype 1: Major Public Program Extension and New Tax Credit

As is the case currently, there would be frequent gaps resulting from job- and family-related transitions. In the absence of periods of guaranteed eligibility, gaps in coverage would also be likely for families whose income fluctuates and is close to the limit for the public program or the tax credit.

Prototype 2: Employer Mandate, Premium Subsidy, and Individual Mandate

To avoid gaps in coverage similar to the current system, it would be necessary to make provisions for smooth transitions of workers from one job to another and in and out of the workforce. Some brief gaps in coverage would be likely given the various potential family- and job-related transitions. Enrollment requirements would need to be relatively simple to minimize those gaps. In addition, there could be discontinuities of plan or provider coverage if an employer changed the plan provided to its workers or as workers changed jobs.

Prototype 3: Individual Mandate and Tax Credit

Under this tax credit strategy, gaps in coverage relating to work or family transitions would be virtually eliminated because the tax credit and mandate would remain with the individual regardless of job, employment, and family

Prototype 2	Prototype 3	Prototype 4
Employer Mandate, Premium Subsidy, and Individual Mandate	Individual Mandate and Tax Credit	Single Payer
Mandatory basic package, more comprehensive at employer's option	Federally defined to reasonably fit amount of tax credit	Comprehensive
"Pay or play" option permitted employers, payroll tax for those not offering coverage	Expanded state regulatory role over small group and nongroup insurance market	Considerable cost sharing at point of service; could enlarge demand for private supplemental coverage

status. Gaps would be more likely to occur if individuals with incomes above the tax credit limit failed to pay the premiums on time, if the credit were not *assignable* to the insurer, or if the family income, size, or dependency changed, making the credit insufficient to support the premium. Monitoring the mandate to prevent gaps during the year might prove challenging after the initial purchase of coverage if the enrollee decided to change plans or his or her economic circumstances changed.

Prototype 4: Single Payer

Once people were enrolled in the single payer system, they would remain so until death, or age 65 if Medicare continued to operate as a separate program. Eligibility would be continuous, with no gaps. Because coverage is not employment based, *portability* through job changes or loss, or family transitions would not be an issue. Family income changes would not trigger eligibility problems either because the entitlement and mandate would reside with the individual and would not be income related, as Medicaid and SCHIP programs are now.

Health Care Coverage Should Be Affordable to Individuals and Families

Prototype 1: Major Public Program Extension and New Tax Credit

Coverage would become more affordable than currently for lower income families that qualify for the expanded public program, for the near-elderly who could buy into Medicare instead of purchasing the more expensive and sometimes unavailable individual policies, and for moderate-income individuals who receive a tax credit. With the design alternative providing a tax credit for lower income as well as moderate-income people, lower income individuals and families would have more choices for coverage, assuming private insurers responded to the demand with attractive and affordable plans. The extent of the benefits, however, would depend on the size of the tax credit. Also, the cost of insurance varies from state to state, depending in part on medical costs in the area, patterns of use, and state regulations and mandates regarding covered services. If those cost differences were not considered in creating the tax credit, the proportion and dollar amount of the remaining premium that would be paid by the individual would vary across the country and could be unaffordable to those in high-cost areas even if generally acceptable nationally. High-risk individuals would be more likely to find a tax credit sufficient to make insurance affordable if the amount of the credit adjusted for age or risk.

The public program would provide comprehensive coverage designed to be affordable for the lower income population. For moderate-income individuals and families, the tax credit would be related progressively to income. Those workers with incomes above that of qualifying for the tax credit would be dependent on what their employer offered for coverage. Employers are currently shifting more insurance costs onto their employees to keep the premium at an acceptable level, and the cost is becoming unaffordable to a growing number of workers (Kaiser/HRET, 2003). Workers and others with income above the level of the tax credit would have the option to purchase coverage in the individual, nongroup market. Without an employer subsidy and individual tax exemption, however, comparable coverage would likely be unaffordable to those without a relatively high income.

Prototype 2: Employer Mandate, Premium Subsidy, and Individual Mandate

Employers would be required to contribute a significant portion of the premium so that the basic package would be affordable to all their workers. The extra premium subsidy for firms with a very low-wage workforce would help make coverage affordable for those workers. The employer could adjust the employee's share of the premium based on individual workers' wages or it could provide a large subsidy on the basic plan to all workers. The availability of large purchasing pools could facilitate decision making for families, but would still have the higher costs associated with the limitations of risk pools in the individual market. The definition of the wage level at which the employer's subsidy would phase out might be set nationally but would need to vary geographically, based on insurance costs variations, in order to assure equitable coverage nationally. Similarly, the subsidy for people purchasing coverage in the individual market or the public program would need to vary across the nation and be sufficient to make the premium affordable for moderate-income families.

Prototype 3: Individual Mandate and Tax Credit

The affordability of coverage to individuals and families depends on the relationship between the size of the tax credit and the cost of premiums relative to family income. Assuming the individual insurance market would respond with policies that fit the size of the tax credit, it is important that the credit amount be large enough to cover a reasonable benefit package. If the services covered are insufficient to meet the needs of the enrollee and he or she has to purchase additional needed services without insurance, this model could become unaffordable for some people. The limitations of tax credits mentioned under the first prototype apply to this model, too.

Because the tax credit would go to lower income as well as moderate-income individuals and would be linked to income, it would be more progressive and equitable than the current tax exemption for employees' health benefits. With a larger population likely to participate in purchasing pools (over which insurers could spread administrative costs and possibly risk, if the pools were very large), some of the higher cost of the individual insurance market could be reduced. However, if that market attracted enough people from employment-based coverage, it could leave employers with the sicker, higher risk workers and increasing premiums.

Because the tax credit would phase out at some specified income level, it would be necessary to define the point at which people are considered wealthy enough to afford the full cost of insurance. If the design alternative to expand regulation of the small group and nongroup insurance market based on national standards were implemented, it could prevent unaffordably high premiums for older people and those with heavy use of health care in the past or medical conditions that are considered risky by insurers. Currently, without federal standards, state regulation is effectively limited by insurers' exit options: insurers can leave a heavily regulated state to do business in less regulated states.

Prototype 4: Single Payer

The main single payer strategy would be readily affordable for most families because it includes only minimal cost sharing and the comprehensive benefit package would reduce the need for additional spending on health services. Nonetheless, those with very low incomes or chronic conditions requiring heavy use might find even minimal cost sharing burdensome. The design alternative that incorporates substantial cost sharing could ultimately distort incentives for appropriate use of services that are built into the benefit structure with variable cost sharing. Substantial cost sharing could induce people to purchase supplemental coverage to reduce or eliminate out-of-pocket costs. Increased cost sharing would be a particular problem for individuals of lower income. The single payer model would require substantial tax revenues. Some individuals or businesses could find the taxes a burden, depending on which taxes were used and their rate and incidence.

Health Insurance Strategy Should Be Affordable and Sustainable for Society

Prototype 1: Major Public Program Extension and New Tax Credit

The expansion of the public programs would be designed with at least some cost sharing. Significantly more cost sharing would be likely in plans purchased with tax credits or offered by employers, so everyone would contribute. The new costs of this strategy would be borne mainly by both the federal government and states through *tax expenditures* and the public program. To the extent that the tax credit was used to contribute to acceptable employment-based plans and extended that coverage, employers would also share in the new costs.

Sustainability: The sustainability of funding for the public program would depend on the sources of revenue used and the long-term cost controls. Utilization controls would depend on actions by each insurer, much as they do now. The tax credit would be a federal tax expenditure. The federal income tax is a relatively sustainable source of revenue; the affordability to society would depend on the amount of the individual credits and aggregate dollars needed. Although costs could be limited in the public programs to some extent, depending on whether the extensions were entitlements or not, the tax credit's budget impact would be like a direct spending program with no spending limits or an entitlement rather than an annual appropriation (Joint Committee on Taxation, 2001). Under this prototype, it would not be possible to limit health care spending in aggregate.

Under the design alternative, the amount of the public subsidy to employers that would be needed to expand workplace coverage would likely need to vary somewhat with the economy. Since 2000 and the economic downturn, smaller firms have been less likely to offer health benefits. The necessary subsidy to employers is likely to be sustainable if employee demand is maintained (Kaiser/HRET, 2003).

Simplicity and Efficiency: The current system is neither efficient nor simple. Although this prototype does not make major changes in the underlying private system, it does make a significant improvement in the public programs by combining them and simplifying the eligibility requirements. The tax credit, while enabling more people to purchase coverage, would likely present recipients with complicated options. The design alternative would give a tax credit to lower income as well as moderate-income families. If they had both the tax credit and the choice of using the public program or private insurance, the operation of the public programs would be somewhat more complex. If the design alternative selected included a tax credit for employers to offer coverage, designing such a program so that it would not penalize those employers already offering and contributing to coverage would also add complexity.

Prototype 2: Employer Mandate, Premium Subsidy, and Individual Mandate

The cost of the federally defined benefit package offered through this prototype would likely be less expensive than current employment-based plans because the mandated coverage would not be as extensive. Employers could choose to offer more extensive benefit packages reflecting the demands of the labor market or their union negotiations. Premiums and cost sharing could be required of all enrollees but kept at a minimal level for those who qualified for the public programs. Administrative factors such as enforcement of the mandate and creation and regulation of purchasing pools would increase administrative costs of the program. The affordability of this system to employers, the main providers of coverage, would depend on how the federal premium subsidy is defined and calculated. Likewise, the size of the employer tax of the design alternative, which permits employers to pay a tax instead of offering coverage, is important. This prototype would rely on employers, who would continue to contribute a substantial portion of the needed revenues.

Sustainability: The sustainability of this insurance strategy would depend to some extent on using revenue sources that could readily increase during difficult economic times when employers might need larger subsidies to provide affordable insurance and the public program would experience an increase in enrollments. The sustainability of the program in the long term would also depend on cost and utilization controls and adjustments to the size of the subsidies. The reduced health costs to state and local governments for uncompensated care, Medicaid, and SCHIP would be significant and have a positive impact on state and local budgets, if no maintenance of effort were required. Under the employer mandate with the "pay or play" design alternative, some firms might drop coverage they currently offer. As a result, their financial support, beyond their tax for not "playing," would be lost to the health system, and possibly to the employees as well if it were not conveyed through a comparable increase in wages or other benefits.

Simplicity and Efficiency: For workers, this prototype would be as easy to use as the current employment-based insurance system. The use of the public programs would be substantially simplified compared to the current situation by combining Medicaid, SCHIP, and the other state coverage programs and by limiting eligibility criteria to family income and lack of private coverage. Health care providers would find this prototype similar to the current system. They would still need to bill many different insurers, and the private insurers would have similar claims processing functions.

This model creates new administrative functions: enforcement of the employer's mandate and calculation of the employer's federal premium subsidy; enforcement of the individual's mandate; and regulation of the private insurance market to ensure the availability of insurance with appropriate basic benefits and operation of the public program. The current functions of the existing private insurance market and its related regulation would remain, and new administrative functions related to the purchasing pools and certification that benefit packages meet federal standards would be added.

The states would have a new role creating and managing large purchasing pools that would make plans available to employers who do not currently offer coverage, including small employer groups, as well as to the self-employed and individuals. The evidence to date does not show that such purchasing arrangements reduce the costs to small employers or pool risks effectively if other group insurance is available with experience-based premiums (Curtis et al., 2001). These arrangements might, however, be more effective when all employers are required to offer coverage and the premium cost is subsidized. Small groups not currently insured, such as small firms, could possibly create a critical mass for the purchasing pools (Wicks, 2002).

Prototype 3: Individual Mandate and Tax Credit

While the dollar values of the individual tax credit could be set within the annual federal budget process, it would function as an entitlement to all those who met the income requirement and would not be subject to a specific congressional appropriation, similar to the tax credit in the first prototype. There would be no limit on aggregate spending on health care, which would depend on individual decisions to purchase insurance and use services, and on the associated costs. There would also be no limit on the aggregate size of the annual federal commitment, but once the credit amount is set, it would not be affected directly by individuals' patterns of service use or providers' charges.

Sustainability: Because the tax credits would be based on the federal income tax, it would be built on the most broadly based tax and it would be a sustainable source. The long-term sustainability of the program, however, would depend on cost controls and adjustments in the subsidy level. It would be difficult to directly impose utilization controls because there would be many independent insurers and even more separate plans.

Simplicity and Efficiency: The elimination of the federal and state public programs along with their confusing eligibility limits and complicated administrative structures would be a significant simplification. This insurance strategy, however, would likely be less efficient than the current system because more people would purchase insurance in the individual and *small-group* market, where administrative and premium costs are highest, and fewer people would obtain coverage through public programs or large employment-based groups, where premiums and administrative costs are lowest. Also, under this tax credit strategy, some employers might be inclined to drop coverage they now provide. Although the individual mandate would mean more healthy people entering the nongroup insurance market, creating a broader risk pool and reducing the *adverse selection* problem of that market as a whole, it would not eliminate the incentive for insurers to "cherry pick" the healthiest people. To the extent that the current limitations of the small group and nongroup insurance markets are ameliorated, particularly under the design alternative, state regulatory and administrative functions become more complicated. However, to the extent that state purchasing pools attract a sufficient portion of purchasers, economies of scale might result.

Choosing their own coverage would not be simple for individuals and families; some education and guidance would be necessary. Also, the individual mandate and tax credit would require the creation of an administrative structure to pay the credit in advance and enforce its appropriate use, both to ensure that people received the correct credit amount and that it was spent on qualified insurance.

Prototype 4: Single Payer

This health insurance strategy would greatly reduce, if not virtually eliminate, employment-based insurance; the small group and nongroup insurance market; current federal, state, and local programs to cover the uninsured; and most out-of-pocket health spending by individuals and families. These major changes potentially create savings for some current participants and significant new public costs, depending on revenue sources used. While there would be substantial public savings resulting from the elimination of the current tax incentives for the purchase of health insurance, they would be balanced by increased tax bills for individuals. Employers' contributions to their employees' health insurance could also be lost to the health system if they were not redirected through a business tax, and lost to the employees if not shifted into the remaining compensation package.

This prototype would create significant labor dislocations in the health insurance and health care industries, although it would likely produce some efficiencies and cost savings for the health sector. Because nearly all health spending would be aggregated under the federal budget, the decision about what society deems affordable would be both very public and unavoidable.

Sustainability: The long-run sustainability of the program would depend on containing cost increases; many potential cost and utilization controls would reside at the federal level. The impact additional cost and utilization controls could have on health access and outcomes is unknown.

The consolidation of spending decisions would have the advantage of placing some federal controls on aggregate health care spending nationally, where it would be subject to taxpayer resistance to tax increases. There would be disadvantages of potentially less consumer pressure to limit spending and problems if the "wrong/inappropriate" level of spending were chosen. It is unclear how, over time, the public's resistance to more taxation would balance against individuals' desires for more and better health services with little out-of-pocket payment. If the funding were predominantly through federal taxes, the system could be politically and economically sustainable, as long as the voting public was willing to support the health care system and balance funding with use to ensure affordability. If the public were unwilling or unable to fund the budget fully, constraints in the form of more limited access to some services could develop over time. Nearly the whole populace would likely contribute both through taxes and cost sharing, but the single payer approach would undoubtedly have significant redistributive effects.

Simplicity and Efficiency: From the perspective of a potential patient, this system would appear simple because eligibility would not change over time nor would reenrollment be required. While procedures and forms that consumers would need to use would be standardized nationally, the simplicity and ease of dealing with a large bureaucracy would likely vary across the country, depending on the contractors and the priority the federal agency placed on consumer education and service.

Single payer systems, such as Medicare, generally are considered to have substantially lower administrative costs than private insurance plans, because the need for advertising, underwriting, and much eligibility and billing work disappears. However, evidence of the specific percentage devoted to administrative costs among all participants in the health system is limited, anecdotal, and insufficient to document the costs of comparable functions.

A single payer strategy could greatly simplify provider billing procedures. There would be no need to determine the secondary health insurers, and standard forms and procedures for all enrollees would make it easier for those submitting bills. On the other hand, additional administrative functions would include a significant increase in federal regulations needed to ensure standards, procedures for updating the benefit package, and payment rates. With only one benefit package, risk selection would not be a concern because there would be little to attract people based on their level of risk to one plan or another. The costs of the healthy and the sick would be averaged across the entire U.S. population.

The supplemental coverage under the design alternative of increased copayments would affect the impact of out-of-pocket cost sharing at the point of service while increasing revenues. One challenge would be determining the level at which cost sharing should be capped for families and individuals so that the copayments would encourage responsible use but not be a deterrent to appropriate use of services, particularly by families with higher than average needs. The level of copayments would require balancing the advantages of cost sharing as a programmatic financing mechanism with the incentives cost sharing creates for the development of supplemental coverage. If the supplemental coverage did more than "wrap around" the public benefit and covered services in the comprehensive package with related amenities and exclusive providers with shorter queues, there would be less control of total spending but additional revenue for the delivery system. With higher cost sharing, it would also be necessary to collect income data and make provision for special no-premium supplemental policies for lower income individuals to avoid inequitable financial barriers to access.

With a single payer system, the federal administrative agency would need to decide how and what to pay for various services and providers. This would present both administrative and political challenges. The planning process as well as negotiations with providers over payments present both the opportunity for greater visibility of the allocation process and the greater risk that the funds and services used would be mismatched.

Health Care Coverage Should Enhance Health and Well-Being by Promoting Access to High-Quality Care That Is Effective, Efficient, Safe, Timely, Patient-Centered, and Equitable

Prototype 1: Major Public Program Extension and New Tax Credit

The combined federal–state public program would include a comprehensive benefit package, comparable to the current Medicaid benefits, which could be designed to promote appropriate, cost-effective use of services even though cost sharing would be minimal for lower income enrollees and have less impact on use. Employment-based insurance and policies purchased on the independent insurance market with the tax credit would meet certain federal standards. There would be a wide variety of benefit packages offered, and with different levels of cost sharing, much as there is today. Cost sharing would be likely to promote appropriate use of services in some but not all plans. The Medicare benefit would be similar to that offered currently.

While the public program could design incentives to promote quality in the health system, at least for its enrollees, its share of provider revenues might be insufficient to induce investment in data systems and other costly improvements. There would be no new requirements on employers or insurers in the private market, so quality improvements would occur to the extent currently expected. If significant numbers of people remain uninsured, the quality of the whole health care system would suffer.

To the extent that health care is inequitably delivered today, particularly disadvantaging members of minority groups due to lack of coverage, this strategy would reduce that inequity by covering more people. This assessment of equity also is applicable to the following three prototypes.

Prototype 2: Employer Mandate, Premium Subsidy, and Individual Mandate

The structure of this prototype would require a federally defined basic benefit package for employment-based coverage and for individually purchased subsidized coverage. It could be defined actuarially or by general benefits to be covered. Some plans might be based on current medical evidence to the extent feasible and designed with cost sharing to promote the use of appropriate services. The required basic benefit package for individual coverage would be less comprehensive than the current average employment-based benefit package, but employers would be allowed to offer richer packages as add-ons to the basic coverage, which some workforces might demand and some labor markets might deliver.

Assuming the more comprehensive employer plans receive the same dollar premium subsidy as the basic plan, lower income workers would be more likely to choose the basic plan. Those workers who could not afford or were not offered a more comprehensive policy might go without needed medical care and suffer poorer health, particularly those with expensive chronic needs. Workers with sufficiently low income who were not eligible for employment-based coverage could qualify for the enriched public program. The design of the public program and the premium assistance to individuals could ensure equitable treatment of employees whether their employer offered benefits or not.

The challenges to promoting quality improvements for clinical as well as administrative management would be similar to the status quo because federal leverage through provider revenues would not be greatly increased. State purchasing pools could also play a role in promoting quality measures. The current incentives for employers to lead in promoting quality would remain. Some progressive employers would continue to pursue quality improvements to the advantage of their employees and the health system. With the employer mandate, the motivation for employers to combine their purchasing activities enough to generate quality improvements and cost savings would be stronger than now.

Prototype 3: Individual Mandate and Tax Credit

The federally defined benefit would be a basic package defined either actuarially or by general benefits with little specificity, much like the previous model. Insurance companies would design their own benefit plans, which might, but would not necessarily, include services proven effective by medical evidence or be designed with cost-sharing incentives for appropriate use. As with the employer mandate prototype, if the size of the tax credit were low relative to the cost of the premium for the basic benefit package, it would be less likely that people could afford a more comprehensive package. They might go without needed care and suffer poorer health if they could not afford to purchase the needed, noncovered services out of pocket. For people with multiple or chronic conditions this might be especially true if there were little regulation of private insurance underwriting practices, because their premiums would be higher than average.

Because all purchases of health care would be through private health insurance companies, mechanisms currently in place through employers and purchasing pools could promote quality improvements in the health system. Individual consumers would be free to switch to plans that they perceived to be of higher quality and collectively could create demand for quality improvements.

Prototype 4: Single Payer

The comprehensive benefit package would be defined nationally and would cover everyone. The cost sharing could be designed to encourage use of services determined to be appropriate and cost effective, but the effect on use might be minimal because the dollar amount of the cost sharing would be minimal. Because this single payer insurance strategy would be comprehensive, the demand for private supplemental insurance might be limited, although anyone who wanted to purchase noncovered services could pay for them out of pocket. Under the design alternative that includes substantially increased cost sharing and supplemental insurance policies, the opportunity for cost sharing to encourage appropriate use would be diminished.

Because the single payer approach could be designed with strong central controls, national quality standards could be defined, imposed, monitored, and reimbursed uniformly and consistently. Whether or not those opportunities were pursued might depend on political forces at the federal level. The development and implementation or enhancement of data systems might prove to be easier and less expensive than currently because systems and reporting standards could be created and imposed at the national level and payments designed to cover capital and operating expenses.

The single payer approach would create a strong incentive to adopt quality measures that would enhance the use of preventive services and cost-effective care because it would reap the benefits of better health and cost savings either in the short or longer term. It would also be uniquely capable of incorporating payment incentives for higher quality care. On the other hand, a strong central bureaucracy could deter creative, innovative quality improvements because of its size, deliberateness, or limitations imposed by Congress. Attempts to set high standards and remove providers that did not meet quality standards would probably meet stronger resistance than in today's Medicare program, because there would be few or no other practice opportunities.

SUMMARY

The assessment of these strategies shows the feasibility of systematically using a body of evidence and a set of principles to guide policy making. The structure of the assessments, based on the principles, gives a straightforward technique to use when designing a new approach. It compares how well the prototypes achieve the principle and highlights which mechanisms are most likely to achieve a particular principle and which strategies might need adjustment. One can also use the assessments to examine an individual prototype by checking its section under each of the five principles. The assessments are summarized in Table 5.2.

By comparing the assessments, one sees that some principles could be achieved better under one model than another. For example, the voluntary approach represented by Prototype 1 is least likely to achieve universal coverage, compared with any of the prototypes incorporating mandates. Each prototype has strengths and weaknesses, achieving some principles more fully than others. All of them offer improvements over the status quo. Some balancing among the objectives emerges: a comprehensive benefit package is more likely both to achieve better health and to cost more than a basic package. If the personal costs of coverage for individuals were reduced, the costs to society would be likely to increase, given a standard benefit package. Although individuals would likely pay for the increased public costs through taxes, there would be a significant shift from current burdens.

The four prototypes were selected to illustrate the broad range of proposals currently circulating and to serve as examples in the preceding analytic exercise. They were described simply, as basic models of each type. It becomes clear in the assessment that each prototype has weaknesses that could be ameliorated through more complex and less "pure" designs. In fact, many proposals under discussion in the public arena take into account some of the limitations highlighted here. The potential to alter a prototype to improve its ability to achieve a specific principle could affect the trade-offs among the principles and could affect the general attractiveness of a particular approach. Not only could the models be improved with further adjustments, but some of the stronger elements in one model could be incorporated into another model. The Committee leaves the debate about the design of a comprehensive, major reform to the public, policy makers, and elected officials. Universal coverage can be achieved if there is political support.

The principles used in the assessment come from the Committee's previous research on the consequences of uninsurance and represent its conclusions on important goals for any strategy to extend coverage. In the next and final chapter the Committee presents its recommendations for extending coverage.

TABLE 5.2 SUMMARY ASSESSMENT OF PROTOTYPES BASED ON COMMITTEE PRINCIPLES

TABLE 5.2 Summary Assessment of Prototypes Based on Committee Principles

Principles	Status Quo	Prototype 1 Major Public Program Extension and New Tax Credit
Coverage should be universal	Not universal; *43 million uninsured*	*Would not achieve universality because voluntary,* but would reduce uninsured population
Coverage should be continuous	*Not continuous;* income, age, family, job, and health-related *gaps in coverage*	Family- and job-related *gaps in coverage*
Coverage should be affordable for individuals and families	*Private coverage unaffordable* to many moderate- and low-income persons	*More affordable than current system* for those with low or moderate income
Strategy should be affordable and sustainable for society	*Not affordable or sustainable for society;* uninsurance is growing; cost of poorer health and shorter lives is $65–$130 billion; some participants contribute; no limit on aggregate health expenditures or on tax expenditures—spending is higher than other countries, sustainability of current public programs depends on economy and political support	All participants contribute; *aggregate expenditures not controlled; new public expenditures for only the public program expansion and tax credit;* sustainability of public program depends on revenue sources and political support; size of credit depends on political support
Coverage should enhance health through high-quality care	*Quality of care* for the population *limited* because one in seven is uninsured	Opportunities to promote quality improvements *similar to current system*

Prototype 2	Prototype 3	Prototype 4
Employer Mandate, Premium Subsidy, and Individual Mandate	Individual Mandate and Tax Credit	Single Payer
Coverage likely to be high; depends on enforcement of mandates	*Depends on size of tax credit, enforcement,* and cost of individual insurance	*Likely to achieve universal coverage*
Brief gaps related to life and job transitions	*Minimal gaps*	*Continuous* until death or age 65
Yes for workers, assuming adequate employer premium assistance; *public program designed to be affordable* for all enrollees	Subsidy based only on income and family size leaves *older, less healthy, and those in expensive areas with less affordable coverage*	*Minimal cost sharing,* but could be problem for lowest income
All participants contribute; *basic package less costly than current employment coverage;* revenue from patients in public program; sustainability depends on revenue sources for employers' premium assistance and public program	No limit on aggregate health expenditures or on tax expenditure, though federal costs relatively predictable and controllable through size of credit; *sustainable through federal income tax base;* size of credit depends on political support	Nearly all participants contribute; *aggregate expenditures controllable,* utilization not directly or centrally controlled; *high cost to federal budget;* administrative savings; sustainability depends on revenue source and political support
Could design quality incentives in expanded public program and basic benefit package; current employer incentives for quality remain	*Similar incentives to current private insurance* system, consumer could choose quality plans	*Potentially yes;* depends on proper design

Vision

The Committee on the Consequences of Uninsurance envisions an approach to health insurance that will promote better overall health for individuals, families, communities, and the nation by providing financial access for everyone to necessary, appropriate, and effective health services.

Principles

1. Health care coverage should be universal.
2. Health care coverage should be continuous.
3. Health care coverage should be affordable to individuals and families.
4. The health insurance strategy should be affordable and sustainable for society.
5. Health care coverage should enhance health and well-being by promoting access to high-quality care that is effective, efficient, safe, timely, patient-centered, and equitable.

Recommendations

The Committee recommends that these principles be used to assess the merits of current proposals and to design future strategies for extending coverage to everyone.

****

The Committee recommends that the President and Congress develop a strategy to achieve universal insurance coverage and establish a firm and explicit schedule to reach this goal by 2010.

****

The Committee recommends that until universal coverage takes effect, the federal and state governments provide resources sufficient for Medicaid and the State Children's Health Insurance Program to cover all persons currently eligible and prevent the erosion of outreach efforts, eligibility, enrollment, and coverage.

6

Conclusions and Recommendations

The charge to the Committee on the Consequences of Uninsurance was "to communicate to the public and policy makers analytical findings about the meaning of a large uninsured population for individuals, families, and their communities, as well as for society as a whole. Its reports should contribute to the public debate about insurance reforms and health care financing." Based on the findings of its first five reports, **the Committee concludes that:**

- **The number of uninsured individuals under age 65 is large, growing, and has persisted despite periods of strong economic growth.**
- **Uninsured children and adults do not receive the care they need; they suffer from poorer health and development, and are more likely to die prematurely than are those with coverage.**
- **Even one uninsured person in a family can put the health and financial stability of the whole family at risk.**
- **When a community has a high uninsured rate, this can adversely affect its overall health status and its health care institutions and providers, and reduce the access of its residents to certain services.**
- **The estimated value across society in healthy years of life gained by providing health insurance coverage to uninsured persons is almost certainly greater than the additional costs of providing those who lack coverage with the same level of services as insured persons use.**

Because having health insurance improves access to appropriate and timely services and access is related to better health, insurance is a key to improving the country's health. The evidence in the Committee's reports on the problems related to uninsurance leads to a logical conclusion—that the interests of our nation and its residents are best served by adopting policies that result in everyone having coverage. Chapter 3 of this report highlights a century of unsuccessful attempts to insure the nation's populace. It also documents efforts that incrementally extended coverage at the federal, state, and county levels. While these efforts have provided insurance for millions of people, they have fallen short. Indeed, more than one of every six Americans under age 65 report they are uninsured for the previous year and the uninsured rate is growing (Mills and Bhandari, 2003). One in three Americans had a period of at least one month without insurance during a two-year period (1996–1997) (Short, 2001). Incremental approaches that are geographically limited, narrowly targeted to a subgroup of the uninsured, temporary, and commit too few new dollars are inadequate to address the problem at hand.

Major reform is needed to make universal coverage a reality. Policy change at the federal level is essential because:

• Federal resources are greater than those available at the state and local levels and can be directed to areas of greatest need.

• Nationwide standards are essential for establishing a uniform minimum level for coverage and benefits, while individual states can provide higher levels if they choose. States are limited by the Employee Retirement Income Security Act of 1974 (ERISA) in their implementation of changes related to employment-based coverage.

Although implementation can be phased in over time, viable reform proposals will need to go beyond the limits of just incremental expansions of existing programs to include an explicit goal and a coherent plan to achieve coverage for everyone, integrated structural changes to correct existing gaps and inefficiencies, and a definite schedule for making measurable progress required to achieve universal coverage within a reasonable timeframe. Most importantly, major reform will require strong, bipartisan political support.

The Committee concludes that universal health insurance coverage for everyone in the United States requires major reform initiated as federal policy.

To facilitate the process of achieving coverage for everyone, the Committee identified principles and policy criteria that can be used to assess the merits of various reform strategies (see Box 6.1). We recognize the essentially political nature of the policy choices that must be made and do not endorse or reject specific reform approaches. The criteria, formulated as Committee principles, are discussed in Chapter 4 and reiterated briefly here.

PRINCIPLES TO GUIDE THE EXTENSION OF COVERAGE

1. Health care coverage should be universal.
2. Health care coverage should be continuous.
3. Health care coverage should be affordable to individuals and families.
4. The health insurance strategy should be affordable and sustainable for society.
5. Health insurance should enhance health and well being by promoting access to high-quality care that is effective, efficient, safe, timely, patient-centered, and equitable.

The Committee recommends that these principles be used to assess the merits of current proposals and to design future strategies for expanding coverage to everyone.

All of the prototypes discussed in Chapter 5 come closer to satisfying the principles than does the status quo. Each could be improved by adjusting various components. Elements from one prototype may be combined with another to maximize the impact or minimize costs. Also, the comprehensiveness of the benefit packages would be weighed against the costs and expected improvements in health. The Committee's intent is not to recommend or reject a particular strategy or to present a specific blueprint, but rather to articulate the principles that should be used to assess various insurance strategies. The Committee believes, however, that the universality principle necessitates an approach that incorporates mandates.

Any proposal for reform inevitably will shift burdens and benefits of health care financing. Depending on the approach selected, those shifts could substantially exceed the actual increase in spending required to cover the uninsured population. While recognizing that financial resources for health care are limited and that shifting current burdens and benefits may be objectionable to those comfortable with the status quo, the Committee believes nonetheless that universal coverage will enhance the overall health and well-being of the nation. Anticipating the political ramifications of the redistributive impacts of a reformed health insurance strategy is beyond the scope of the Committee's charge. The inevitability of such shifts is not a reason for inaction. We must acknowledge the need to restructure health care finance fundamentally in order to extend coverage to everyone.

Significant new public policies will be necessary to address the issue of uninsurance. Additional public resources to finance insurance will be needed as well, although these may be reduced or offset by savings elsewhere. The Committee recognizes that the American public in the past has been reluctant to support coverage for the uninsured because it would likely entail additional taxes or a major shifting of budgetary resources. A more complete understanding of the great costs we are incurring as a society because of the lack of universal coverage might overcome this reluctance. Although some of the existing payments for care for the uninsured might be shifted into a new, comprehensive program, we also recognize that it is highly unlikely that all current expenditures would become available to support a new program.

The Committee recognizes that a program of universal coverage will take time to develop, adopt, and implement. The political and administrative complexities and financing challenges of implementing even the simplest model should not be underestimated. The Committee therefore urges that planning, including an aggressive timetable, begin immediately, with the goal of universal coverage by 2010. The Committee is optimistic that the task is achievable by this date and that it is a reasonable target. This date is consistent with the federal government's Healthy People 2010 initiative to increase the years and quality of life nationally and eliminate disparities in health among population groups (DHHS, 2000). The first objective of the initiative's Access to Health Care goal is to increase the proportion of the population under age 65 that has health care coverage; the target is 100 percent coverage by 2010 (DHHS, 2000).

Like any major tax law or other social program reform, transitions for large and even small changes in health care finance can be costly. Any plan for phasing in universal coverage should recognize that change in the current health insurance system will be complex and potentially confusing. Thus, the coherence and simplicity of a minimal number of transitional stages are important goals for a phase-in strategy.

The Committee recommends that the President and Congress develop a strategy to achieve universal insurance coverage and establish a firm and explicit schedule to reach this goal by 2010.

Because full insurance coverage for the whole population will take time to achieve, several actions should be taken to prevent further erosion of existing public insurance programs. During the current economic downturn, many states and municipalities are experiencing reduced revenues. This fiscal crisis is intensified by rising health care costs and insurance premiums and by growing numbers of unemployed residents who are uninsured and eligible for public coverage (Smith et al., 2003). As a result of budget shortfalls in 2002, many states are planning significant cutbacks in the State Children's Health Insurance Program (SCHIP) and their Medicaid program, which is the second largest line item in most states' operating budgets (Schneider, 2002; KCMU, 2003b). Generally, those cutbacks had not been implemented by April 2003, but future cuts are anticipated (KCMU, 2003c). With 50 million nonelderly persons enrolled in Medicaid and another 5.3 million in SCHIP, it is important to assure funds for continued coverage and to expand enrollment in periods when more people meet existing eligibility criteria (CMS, 2003a; KCMU, 2003a). It is also important to remember that the original authorization and appropriation for the SCHIP program was limited to 10 years and is due to expire in 2007. Provisions for its continuation will be necessary if the reform strategy is not fully implemented by that date. Otherwise, the population served by the current program will become uninsured.

The Committee recognizes the current economic pressures on all levels of government. More enrollees will require additional funds. An estimated 3 million lower income adults are currently eligible but not enrolled in Medicaid, representing 16 percent of all lower income adults (Schneider, 2002). Another 4.3 million children are eligible for Medicaid or SCHIP, but not enrolled (Kenney et al., 2003). If these people were covered by the existing programs, the uninsured population would be significantly reduced. Getting people enrolled in these public programs is necessary but not sufficient; keeping them in the program is also important. Medicaid can be difficult to obtain and hard to keep. While most states have implemented administrative changes to facilitate enrollment, in the face of serious budget constraints some states have taken steps to curtail outreach efforts, limit eligibility of parents, and rescind 12-month continuous eligibility for children (Ross and Cox, 2003). Efforts should be taken to reduce the number of people without coverage because of complex enrollment procedures and administrative barriers or obstacles.

Individuals earning less than the poverty level are particularly likely to lose health insurance, whether public or private. About 19 percent of children and 17 percent of adults who are covered by Medicaid at the start of the year lose that coverage during the year, even though many remain eligible (Ku and Ross, 2002). Among low-income people with private coverage, 13 percent of children and adults who start the year with coverage lose it before the end of the year. Continuous coverage for those who are intermittently insured could reverse some of the negative consequences of uninsurance. While many states have provided outreach and streamlined enrollment and reenrollment procedures for SCHIP, there has not been as much progress in the Medicaid program, for which two-thirds of uninsured children are eligible.

The Committee recommends that until universal coverage takes effect, the federal and state governments provide resources sufficient for Medicaid and SCHIP to cover all persons currently eligible and prevent the erosion of outreach efforts, eligibility, enrollment, and coverage.

The public coverage programs are critical for those who *otherwise would be uninsured*. For those who *currently are uninsured*, it is important to maintain the existing capacity of health care institutions and providers who often make needed services available. The disruptions of transition to universal coverage for those providers and institutions should be minimized. The Committee also recognizes that problems of access to health care will remain in some geographic areas and for certain populations. Insurance coverage will reduce but not eliminate the need to support service capacity in certain underserved areas and for particular underserved populations.

The Committee believes we all have a stake in *how* these recommendations are implemented as well as *whether or not* they are implemented. Currently all Americans bear the costs of a sizable uninsured population:

- the ill health, impaired development, and early deaths of the uninsured, measured as the lost value of healthy life years;
- much of the costs of care provided to the uninsured;
- the financial instability of all families with at least one uninsured member;
- the negative impact on health care institutions and on the communities they serve; and
- the diminution of democratic cultural and political values of equal respect and equal opportunity.

Doing nothing to change current policies carries substantial costs which will continue to grow in the future as health services become increasingly effective. Indeed, the underlying purpose of the Committee's project has been to identify and increase awareness of the consequences associated with uninsurance, in the belief that an informed public will generate public policies to ameliorate the problem. The next steps require bipartisan political action at the federal level to move the process forward. Box 6.2 reminds us that this peculiarly American dilemma of health insurance reform has been with us a long time. Even more importantly, it reminds us of why we should delay reforms no longer.

BOX 6.2
A Page from History

The following text is from President Richard Nixon's conclusion of his Special Message to Congress, February 18, 1971, in which he transmitted his proposal for health insurance reform.

"It is health which is real wealth," said Gandhi, "and not pieces of gold and silver." That statement applies not only to the lives of men but also to the life of nations. And nations, like men, are judged in the end by the things they hold most valuable.

Not only is health more important than economic wealth, it is also its foundation. It has been estimated, for example, that ten percent of our country's economic growth in the past half century has come because a declining death rate has produced an expanded labor force.

Our entire society, then, has a direct stake in the health of every member. In carrying out its responsibilities in this field, a nation serves its own best interests, even as it demonstrates the breadth of its spirit and the depth of its compassion.

Yet we cannot truly carry out these responsibilities unless the ultimate focus of our concern is the personal health of the individual human being. We dare not get so caught up in our systems and our strategies that we lose sight of *his* needs or compromise *his* interests. We can build an effective National Health Strategy only if we remember the central truth that the only way to serve our people well is to better serve each person.

The Committee has demonstrated that through both good economic times and bad and despite decades of efforts to implement universal health insurance coverage, the United States has continued to have a large and growing uninsured population. Although there was a slight dip in the number uninsured in 1999 following several years of prosperous economic conditions, it was so small and temporary that it is clear that economic growth alone will not eliminate the presence of a large uninsured population. That population, because of lack of insurance, has experienced less or no access to needed health care. The benefits of universal coverage would enrich all Americans, whether accounted for in terms of improved health and longer life spans, greater economic productivity, financial security, or the stabilization of communities' health care systems. We all benefit as well because health insurance contributes essentially to obtaining the kind and quality of health care that can express the equality and dignity of every person. Unless we can ensure universal coverage, we fail as a nation to deliver the great promise of our health care system, as well as of the values we live by as a society. **It is time for our nation to extend coverage to everyone.**

A

Data Tables

TABLE A.1 Federal Poverty Guidelines, 2002 and 2003

Family Size in 48 Contiguous States	Federal Poverty Level (FPL)						
	FPL for 2002			FPL for 2003			
	100% FPL	200% FPL	300% FPL	100% FPL	200% FPL	300% FPL
1 person	$8,860	$17,720	$26,580	$8,980	$17,960	$26,940
2 persons	$11,940	$23,880	$35,820	$12,120	$24,240	$36,360
3 persons	$15,020	$30,040	$45,060	$15,260	$30,520	$45,780
4 persons	$18,100	$36,200	$54,300	$18,400	$36,800	$55,200

SOURCE: DHHS, 2003.

TABLE A.2 Distribution of Uninsured Population and Probabilities of Going Without Coverage by Selected Characteristics, 2002

	No. in Population (thousands)	Distribution in Population (%)	No. of Uninsured (est.) (thousands)	Uninsured Rate (%)
Total	285,933	100.0	43,574	15.2
Work experience (18-64 yrs old)				
Total	178,388	100.0	34,785	19.5
Worked during year	142,918	80.1	25,679	18.0
Worked full-time	118,411	66.4	19,911	16.8
Worked part-time	24,506	13.7	5,767	23.5
Did not work during year	35,470	19.9	9,106	25.7
Household income (not income for health insurance unit)				
Less than $25,000	62,979	22.0	14,776	23.5
$25,000 to $49,999	75,927	26.6	14,638	19.3
$50,000 to $74,999	58,622	20.5	6,904	11.8
$75,000 or more	88,406	30.9	7,256	8.2
Federal poverty level				
Total (in poverty universe[a])	285,317	100.0	43,371	15.2
Earning up to 100% FPL	34,570	12.1	10,492	30.4
Earning between 100% and 200% FPL	12,514	4.4	3,488	27.9
Educational attainment (18 years and older)				
Total	212,622	100.0	35,042	16.5
No high school diploma	34,829	16.4	9,768	28.0
High school graduate only	67,512	31.8	12,671	18.8
Some college, no degree	41,319	19.4	6,214	15.0
Associate degree	16,350	7.7	1,981	12.1
Bachelor's degree or higher	52,612	24.7	4,408	8.4
Firm size (18-64 yrs old)				
Total	142,918	100.0	25,679	18.0
Less than 25 employees	42,025	29.4	12,520	29.8
25 to 99 employees	18,650	13.0	3,686	19.8
100 to 499 employees	19,579	13.7	2,626	13.4
500 to 999 employees	7,705	5.4	812	10.5
1000 or more employees	54,958	38.4	6,035	11.0
Age				
Under 18 years	73,312	25.6	8,531	11.6
18 to 24 years	27,438	9.6	8,128	29.6
25 to 34 years	39,243	13.7	9,769	24.9
35 to 44 years	44,074	15.4	7,781	17.7
45 to 54 years	40,234	14.1	5,586	13.9
55 to 64 years	27,399	9.6	3,521	12.8
65 years or more	34,234	12.0	258	0.8

Continued

TABLE A.2 Continued

	No. in Population (thousands)	Distribution in Population (%)	No. of Uninsured (est.) (thousands)	Uninsured Rate (%)
Immigrant and nativity status				
Born in United States	252,463	88.3	32,388	12.8
Foreign born	33,471	11.7	11,186	33.4
Naturalized citizen	12,837	4.5	2,251	17.5
Noncitizen	20,634	7.2	8,935	43.3
Race and ethnicity				
White, alone or in combination	235,036	82.2	33,320	14.2
African American, alone or in combination	37,350	13.1	7,429	19.9
Hispanic, all combinations	39,384	13.8	12,756	32.4
Asian/S. Pacific Islander, alone or in combination	12,504	4.4	2,248	18.0
Gender				
Male	139,876	48.9	23,327	16.7
Female	146,057	51.1	20,246	13.9
Census region of residence				
Northeast	54,139	18.9	7,057	13.0
Midwest	64,581	22.6	7,533	11.7
South	101,800	35.6	17,773	17.5
West	65,413	22.9	11,210	17.1

[a]The U.S. Census Bureau uses the concept of poverty universe to describe all respondents for whom information about income is available.

NOTE: Fractions may not add to 100 percent because of rounding, because some people may report coverage from more than one source during the course of a year, and because respondents may fall into more than one reporting category, for example, in the case of race and ethnicity.

SOURCES: Mills and Bhandari, 2003; U.S. Census Bureau, 2003a,b,c.

TABLE A.3 DISTRIBUTION OF UNINSURED POPULATION UNDER AGE 65 AND PROBABILITIES OF GOING WITHOUT COVERAGE, BY STATE OF RESIDENCE, 2002

TABLE A.3 Distribution of Uninsured Population Under Age 65 and Probabilities of Going Without Coverage, by State of Residence, 2002

	No. in Population (thousands)	Distribution in Population (%)	No. of Uninsured (est.) (thousands)	Distribution of Uninsured (%)	Uninsured Rate (%)
U.S. total	251,700	100.0	43,316	100.0	17.2
Alabama	3,820	1.5	564	1.3	14.8
Alaska	588	0.2	117	0.3	20.0
Arizona	4,713	1.9	913	2.1	19.4
Arkansas	2,311	0.9	438	1.0	18.9
California	31,732	12.6	6,361	14.7	20.0
Colorado	4,033	1.6	717	1.7	17.8
Connecticut	2,885	1.1	355	0.8	12.3
Delaware	701	0.3	79	0.2	11.2
District of Columbia	504	0.2	73	0.2	14.5
Florida	13,675	5.4	2,816	6.5	20.6
Georgia	7,683	3.1	1,354	3.1	17.6
Hawaii	1,059	0.4	121	0.3	11.4
Idaho	1,151	0.5	233	0.5	20.2
Illinois	11,052	4.4	1,758	4.1	15.9
Indiana	5,362	2.1	794	1.8	14.8
Iowa	2,523	1.0	274	0.6	10.9
Kansas	2,346	0.9	280	0.6	11.9
Kentucky	3,526	1.4	546	1.3	15.5
Louisiana	3,914	1.6	814	1.9	20.8
Maine	1,073	0.4	144	0.3	13.4
Maryland	4,838	1.9	725	1.7	15.0
Massachusetts	5,615	2.2	637	1.5	11.3
Michigan	8,828	3.5	1,152	2.7	13.1
Minnesota	4,519	1.8	397	0.9	8.8
Mississippi	2,482	1.0	464	1.1	18.7
Missouri	4,905	1.9	646	1.5	13.2
Montana	774	0.3	139	0.3	17.9
Nebraska	1,492	0.6	173	0.4	11.6
Nevada	1,873	0.7	417	1.0	22.3
New Hampshire	1,116	0.4	125	0.3	11.2
New Jersey	7,470	3.0	1,181	2.7	15.8
New Mexico	1,594	0.6	385	0.9	24.2
New York	16,860	6.7	3,014	7.0	17.9
North Carolina	7,162	2.8	1,362	3.1	19.0
North Dakota	545	0.2	69	0.2	12.7
Ohio	9,892	3.9	1,331	3.1	13.5
Oklahoma	3,022	1.2	600	1.4	19.9
Oregon	3,106	1.2	511	1.2	16.5

TABLE A.3 Continued

	No. in Population (thousands)	Distribution in Population (%)	No. of Uninsured (est.) (thousands)	Distribution of Uninsured (%)	Uninsured Rate (%)
Pennsylvania	10,359	4.1	1,377	3.2	13.3
Rhode Island	914	0.4	104	0.2	11.3
South Carolina	3,453	1.4	496	1.1	14.4
South Dakota	651	0.3	84	0.2	13.0
Tennessee	5,054	2.0	606	1.4	12.0
Texas	19,403	7.7	5,515	12.7	28.4
Utah	2,129	0.8	305	0.7	14.3
Vermont	543	0.2	66	0.2	12.2
Virginia	6,329	2.5	962	2.2	15.2
Washington	5,385	2.1	848	2.0	15.7
West Virginia	1,468	0.6	254	0.6	17.3
Wisconsin	4,838	1.9	535	1.2	11.0
Wyoming	430	0.2	86	0.2	20.0

SOURCE: U.S. Census Bureau, 2003d.

TABLE A.4 Summary of National Surveys Compiling Information on Health Insurance Status of the Population (Estimates for Population Under Age 65)

Survey and Sponsor	Frequency of Survey	Sample
Community Tracking Study, Household Survey—Center for Studying Health System Change	Two-year cycle for first three rounds (1996–1997, 1998–1999, 2000–2001); fourth round in 2003	32,000 households; 60,000 individuals in survey
Current Population Survey— U.S. Census Bureau	Annual; health insurance-related questions since 1980	80,000 households; 130,000 individuals
National Health Interview Survey —National Center for Health Statistics, Centers for Disease Control and Prevention	Annual; health insurance questions made part of each year's survey since 1997	43,000 households containing 106,000 individuals
National Survey of America's Families—Urban Institute	First conducted in 1997, subsequent rounds in 1999 and 2002	44,000 households with 106,000 individuals

Methods	Who Counts As "Uninsured"	Estimated Uninsured and Period Uninsured
Telephone survey of nationally representative sample in 60 randomly selected metropolitan statistical areas (MSAs); more intensive sampling in 12 of these MSAs	Individuals reporting no insurance type asked to verify that they are uninsured	2000–2001 33.8 million uninsured; uninsured at time of interview (Cunningham, 2003)
National probability sample with independent state-level samples allowing for state-level estimates. Telephone and face-to-face interviews. One person answers on behalf of household members	Individuals reporting no insurance type asked to verify that they are uninsured	2002 43.3 million; uninsured throughout prior calendar year (Mills and Bhandari, 2003)
National probability sample with in-person interviews with each family as a group	Individuals reporting no insurance type asked to verify that they are uninsured	2002 40.0 million; uninsured at time of interview (CDC, 2003)
Telephone survey of nationally representative sample of persons under 65, also representative for 13 states, with in-person interviews of a sample of households without telephones	Individuals reporting no insurance type asked to verify that they are uninsured	1999 36 million uninsured; uninsured at time of interview (Haley and Zuckerman, 2003)

Continued

TABLE A.4 Continued

Survey and Sponsor	Frequency of Survey	Sample
Panel surveys		
Medical Expenditure Panel Survey—Agency for Healthcare Research and Quality	New in 1996; new panel annually. Comparable prior surveys: National Medical Expenditure Survey, 1987; National Medical Care Expenditure Survey, 1977	32,122 persons in 2001 Household Component
Survey of Income and Program Participation—U.S. Census Bureau	New panel every 2–4 years since 1983. Monthly data based on quarterly interviews	36,700 households in 2001 panel

Methods	Who Counts As "Uninsured"	Estimated Uninsured and Period Uninsured
National probability sample. Six interviews over 30 months. Computer-assisted in-person and telephone interviews	Residual—persons not reporting any type of coverage	2001 31.3 million uninsured throughout calendar year, 61.9 million uninsured at any time during the year; reports provide status during a reference period of 3–5 months; data allow for monthly analysis (Rhoades and Cohen, 2003)
In-person interviews with each household member over age 15; adults asked about children	Residual—persons not reporting any type of coverage	1998 21.1 million uninsured throughout calendar year, 56.8 million uninsured at any time during the year; months combined for annual estimate (Congressional Budget Office, 2003)

B

Glossary and Acronyms

Adverse Selection The disproportionate enrollment of individuals with poorer than average health expectations in certain health plans. Over time, as plan premiums rise as a result of higher enrollee health care costs, the plan becomes less attractive to relatively healthy potential enrollees, disproportionately attracting relatively sicker enrollees in successive enrollment cycles, which results in spiraling costs.

Affinity Group A group of people with a common organizational interest or membership, other than for the purchase of health insurance, for example, membership in a professional society.

Benefit The particular services covered by a health plan and the amount payable for a loss under a specific insurance coverage (indemnity benefits) or as the guarantee of payment for certain services (service benefits).

Charity Care Generally, physician and hospital services provided to persons who are unable to pay for services, especially those who are low income, uninsured, and underinsured. A high proportion of the costs of charity care is derived from services for children and pregnant women (e.g., neonatal intensive care).*

---

*Adapted from the Academy for Health Services Research and Health Policy glossary at: http://www.academyhealth.org/publications.glossary.pdf. Accessed February 4, 2002.

Coinsurance The percentage of a covered medical expense that a beneficiary must pay, after any required deductible is met.

Community Rating Calculating premiums based on the average costs of all of an insurer's subscribers rather than on the experience of a subgroup or of individuals.

Copayment A fixed payment per service (e.g., $15 per office visit or procedure) paid by a health plan member.

Cost Sharing The portion of health care expenses that a health plan member must pay directly, including deductibles, copayments, and coinsurance, but not including the premium.

Cost Shifting Transfer of health care provider costs that are not reimbursed by one payer to other payers through higher charges for services.

Cross-Subsidization Payments made for services rendered to one individual or group that are used to cover shortfalls in individual payments for services rendered to another individual or group.

Crowd-Out, Substitution A phenomenon whereby new public programs or expansions of existing public programs designed to extend coverage to the uninsured prompt some privately insured persons to drop their private coverage and take advantage of the expanded public subsidy.*

Deductible The amount of loss or expense that must be incurred by an insured or otherwise covered individual before an insurer will assume any liability for all or part of the remaining cost of covered services. Deductibles may be either fixed-dollar amounts or the value of specified services (such as 2 days of hospital care or one physician visit). Deductibles are usually tied to some reference period over which they must be incurred (e.g., $100 per calendar year, benefit period, or spell of illness).*

Dependent An insured's spouse (not legally separated from the insured) and unmarried child(ren) who meet certain eligibility requirements and are not otherwise insured under the same group policy. The precise definition of a dependent varies by insurer or employer.

Disproportionate Share Adjustment, Hospital (DSH) A payment adjustment under Medicare's prospective payment system or under Medicaid for hospitals that serve a relatively large volume of low-income patients.*

Entitlement A legal obligation on the federal government to make payments to a person, business, or unit of government that meets the criteria set in law. Congress generally controls entitlement programs by setting eligibility criteria and benefit or payment rules—not by providing budget authority in the appropriation act (CBO, 2002).

Equity Concerning fairness and justice, the idea of balancing legitimate, competing claims of individuals in society in a way that is seen as impartial or disinterested. Distributional equity, which concerns the fair distribution of some good or service of interest, has been the dominant equity concern both of normative economic analysis and of health policy makers (Hurley, 2000).

Experience Rating Setting health insurance premiums based in whole or in part on past claims history of a particular group or its anticipated future claims.

Federal Poverty Level (FPL) One of two federal poverty measurements; also known as "poverty guidelines." Issued annually in the *Federal Register* by the U.S. Department of Health and Human Services; it applies to persons of all ages in family units. The guidelines are a simplification of the poverty measurements for administrative purposes, such as determining financial eligibility for certain federal programs. In 2003, the FPL for a family unit of one was $8,980; for a family unit of three, $15,260; and for a family unit of four, $18,400 (see Appendix A, Table A.1) (DHHS, 2003).

Fee-for-Service An approach to billing for health services in which providers charge a separate price or fee for each service provided or patient encounter. Under fee-for-service, the level of expenditures for health care depends on both the levels at which fees are set and the number and types of services provided.★

Global Budget A budget set in advance to contain costs among a group of hospitals, where each hospital accepts an aggregate cap on its annual revenues.★

Gross Domestic Product (GDP) The total market value of goods and services produced domestically during a given period. The components of GDP are consumption (both household and government), gross investment (both private and government), and net exports (CBO, 2002).

Guaranteed Issue Insurance coverage that does not require the insured to provide evidence of insurability. Alternatively, it is the requirement that insurers offer coverage to groups or individuals during some period each year.★

Health Capital The present value of a person's health over the course of their lifetime (Cutler and Richardson, 1997).

Health-Related Quality of Life A research construct developed by the Centers for Disease Control and Prevention to help monitor progress in achieving national health objectives. Its core element consists of four questions that encompass general self-reported health status, the number of unhealthy days within a recent time period (e.g., the month before the interview) for both physical and mental dimensions, and restricted activity days.

High-Risk Pool A subsidized health insurance pool organized by a state as a subsidized alternative for individuals who have been denied health insurance because of a medical condition or whose premiums are rated significantly higher than the average due to health status or claims experience. It is commonly operated through an association composed of all health insurers in a state. The Health Insurance Portability and Accountability Act allows states to use high-risk pools as an "acceptable alternative mechanism" that satisfies the statutory requirements for ensuring access to health insurance coverage for certain individuals.

Individual Market, Nongroup Market The insurance market for products sold to individuals rather than to members of groups. Typically each state regulates its own nongroup market.

Integrated Delivery System, Integrated Services Network A group of health care providers and institutions that delivers services across the continuum of care to a target population and is accountable for the financial and clinical outcomes of the services delivered.★

Job Lock A distortion in job mobility attributed to employer-provided health insurance when employees keep jobs they would rather leave for fear of losing coverage (from Madrian, 1994).

Maintenance of Effort The requirement that states, local governments, employers, individuals, or other organizations continue spending their own funds at previous levels to support a particular purpose or program after reform.

Medical Savings Account A vehicle through which individuals can accumulate funds to pay for health care or insurance premiums, subject to federal income taxation but tax exempt in some states.★

Medical Underwriting An insurance practice of determining whether to accept or refuse individuals or groups for insurance coverage (or to adjust coverage or premiums) on the basis of an assessment of the risk they pose and other criteria (e.g., insurer's business objectives).

Nongroup Market See definition for individual market.

Out-of-Pocket Expenses Payments made by an individual or family for medical services that are not reimbursed by health insurance. They can include payments for health plan deductibles, coinsurance, services not covered by the plan, provider charges in excess of the plan's limits, and enrollee premium payments.

Portability of Benefits A guarantee of continuous coverage without waiting periods (e.g., for a preexisting health condition) for persons moving between plans.★

Preexisting Condition A physical or mental condition that exists prior to the effective date of health insurance coverage.

Premium, Total The purchase price of a health insurance policy. **Out-of-Pocket Premium** or **Employee Share** Most workers enrolled in employment-based policies do not pay the total premium for their coverage but only a part of it, with the remainder subsidized by the employer. **Risk-Adjusted Premium** The price or amount of the premium reflects the expected utilization of the policy holder or group of enrolled persons and thus the financial liability for the insurer, often estimated according to the gender, age, and health status of the insured.

Purchasing Pool A group of people who purchase health insurance jointly.

Quality of Care The degree to which health services for individuals and populations increase the likelihood of desired health outcomes and are consistent with current professional knowledge (IOM, 1990).

Reinsurance The spreading of the costs to an insurer of underwriting health insurance coverage by reselling insurance products in the secondary market.★

Risk Pool A group of people whose actuarial risk is considered together.

Self-Insurance Funding of medical care expenses, generally by an employer, in whole or part through internal resources rather than through transfer of risk to an insurer.

Small-Group Market The insurance market for products sold to groups that are smaller than a specified size, typically employer groups. The size of groups included usually depends on state insurance laws and thus varies from state to state, with 50 employees the most common size.★

Social Insurance Old-age, disability, health, or other insurance that is mandated by statute for defined categories of individuals or the entire population, usually financed by payroll and other taxes.

Spillover Effect A direct effect, either positive or negative, on a person's or institution's welfare or profit developing as a byproduct of some other person's or firm's activity. Also referred to as an economic externality.

Supplemental Coverage In the case of Medicare, private health insurance designed to cover expenses not paid for by Medicare, often designated as Medigap policies.

Tax Credit, Refundable, Advanceable, Assignable An amount subtracted from the tax bill to be paid (tax liability). In contrast to a credit, an exemption subtracts some amount from income on which the tax is computed. If the credit is refundable, the taxpayer should receive a refund for the amount by which the credit exceeds the tax liability. An advanceable credit can be used by the taxpayer for up to a year before the filing date for taxes, for example, to subsidize monthly premium payments. An assignable credit can be used by the taxpayer to direct payment of the credit to another party, for example, to an insurer as a premium payment.

Tax Expenditure The loss of federal tax revenue due to a special exclusion, exemption, or deduction from gross income in federal tax law, the provision of a special credit or a preferential tax rate, or a deferral of tax liability (U.S. Congress, 1974).

Tax Incidence The distribution of the final burden of taxation across a population, taking into account all shifts in tax payments, for example, the shift in tax burden from a producer of goods to the consumer by means of a higher price for the goods.

Uncompensated Care Service provided by physicians and hospitals for which no payment is received from the patient or from third-party payers. Some costs of these services may be covered through cost shifting. Not all uncompensated care results from charity care. It also includes bad debts from persons who are not classified as charity cases, but who are unable or unwilling to pay their bills.★

ACRONYMS

AALL   American Association for Labor Legislation

COBRA   Consolidated Omnibus Budget Reconciliation Act of 1985

EMTALA   Emergency Medical Treatment and Labor Act of 1986

ERISA   Employee Retirement Income Security Act of 1974

FPL   Federal Poverty Level (see Appendix A, Table A.1)

HIPAA   Health Insurance Portability and Accountability Act of 1996

SCHIP   State Children's Health Insurance Program

TA   Trade Act of 2002

C

Biographical Sketches

COMMITTEE ON THE CONSEQUENCES OF UNINSURANCE
SUBCOMMITTEE ON STRATEGIES AND MODELS FOR PROVIDING HEALTH INSURANCE

Mary Sue Coleman, Ph.D., *Co-chair,* is president of the University of Michigan. She is professor of biological chemistry in the University of Michigan Medical School and professor of chemistry in the College of Literature, Science and the Arts. She previously was president of the University of Iowa and president of the University of Iowa Health Systems (1995–2002). Dr. Coleman served as provost and vice president for academic affairs at the University of New Mexico (1993–1995) and dean of research and vice chancellor at the University of North Carolina at Chapel Hill (1990–1992). For 19 years, she was both faculty member and Cancer Center administrator at the University of Kentucky in Lexington, where her research focused on the immune system and malignancies. Dr. Coleman is a member of the Institute of Medicine (IOM) and a fellow of the American Association for the Advancement of Science and of the American Academy of Arts and Sciences. She serves on the Life Sciences Corridor Steering Committee for the State of Michigan, the Executive Committee of the American Association of Universities, and other voluntary advisory bodies and corporate boards.

Arthur L. Kellermann, M.D., M.P.H., *Co-chair,* is professor and director, Center for Injury Control, Rollins School of Public Health, Emory University, and professor and chairman, Department of Emergency Medicine, School of

Medicine, Emory University. Dr. Kellermann has served as principal investigator or co-investigator on several research grants, including federally funded studies of handgun-related violence and injury, emergency cardiac care, and the use of emergency room services. Among many awards and distinctions, he is a fellow of the American College of Emergency Physicians (1992), is the recipient of a meritorious service award from the Tennessee State Legislature (1993) and the Hal Jayne Academic Excellence Award from the Society for Academic Emergency Medicine (1997), and was elected to membership in the Institute of Medicine (1999). In addition, Dr. Kellermann is a member of the editorial board of the journal *Annals of Emergency Medicine*, and has served as a reviewer for the *New England Journal of Medicine*, the *Journal of the American Medical Association*, and the *American Journal of Public Health*.

Ronald M. Andersen, Ph.D., is the Fred W. and Pamela K. Wasserman Professor of Health Services and professor of sociology at the University of California at Los Angeles School of Public Health. He teaches courses in health services organization, research methods, evaluation, and leadership. Dr. Andersen received his Ph.D. in sociology at Purdue University. He has studied access to medical care for his entire professional career of 30 years. Dr. Andersen developed the Behavioral Model of Health Services Use that has been used extensively nationally and internationally as a framework for utilization and cost studies of general populations as well as special studies of minorities, low-income populations, children, women, the elderly, the homeless, the HIV-positive population, and oral health. He has directed three national surveys of access to care and has led numerous evaluations of local and regional populations and programs designed to promote access to medical care. Dr. Andersen's other research interests include international comparisons of health services systems, graduate medical education curricula, physician health services organization integration, and evaluations of geriatric and primary care delivery. He is a member of the Institute of Medicine and was on the founding board of the Association for Health Services Research. He has been chair of the Medical Sociology Section of the American Sociological Association. In 1994 he received the association's Leo G. Reeder Award for Distinguished Service to Medical Sociology; in 1996 he received the Distinguished Investigator Award from the Association for Health Services Research; and in 1999 he received the Baxter Allegiance Health Services Research Prize.

John Z. Ayanian, M.D., M.P.P., is associate professor of medicine and health care policy at Harvard Medical School and Brigham and Women's Hospital, where he practices general internal medicine. His research focuses on quality of care and access to care for major medical conditions, including colorectal cancer and myocardial infarction. He has extensive experience in the use of cancer registries to assess outcomes and evaluate the quality of cancer care. In addition, he has studied the effects of race and gender on access to kidney transplants and on quality of care for other medical conditions. Dr. Ayanian is deputy editor of the journal *Medical Care*, director of the general internal medicine fellowship at Brigham and Women's Hospital, and a fellow of the American College of Physicians.

Patricia Butler, J.D., Dr.P.H.,★ is a self-employed policy analyst who works on issues of health care financing, delivery, and regulation on behalf of state legislative and executive branch officials. She has been a member of the National Academy for State Health Policy since its inception in 1987 and serves on the editorial advisory board of the Bureau of National Affairs' *Pension & Benefits Reporter*. Dr. Butler received her B.A. from the University of California (UC) in 1966, her law degree from UC Berkeley's Boalt Hall School of Law in 1969, and her doctorate in health policy from the University of Michigan's School of Public Health in 1996. She has published in-depth analyses of ERISA and other legal issues in health policy.

Sheila P. Davis, B.S.N., M.S.N., Ph.D., is professor in the School of Nursing at the University of Mississippi Medical Center. She is also vice president of Davis, Davis & Associates, a health maintenance consultant company. Her research focuses on minority health issues, especially cardiovascular risk among ethnic populations. Dr. Davis is the founder and chair of the Cardiovascular Risk Reduction in Children Committee at the University of Mississippi. This is a multidisciplinary committee committed to reducing cardiovascular risks in children. Dr. Davis is a member of the American Nurses Association and has written numerous publications on the profession and the experiences of ethnic minorities in the health professions. She is author of a faith-based program, Healthy Kid's Seminar, which is used to promote adoption of healthy lifestyle choices by children. Dr. Davis serves on the editorial review board of the *Journal of Cultural Diversity* and the *Association of Black Nursing Faculty Journal*. She is also founder and editor in chief of the *Online Journal of Health Ethics*.

George C. Eads, Ph.D.,★ is vice president of Charles River Associates (CRA), Washington, D.C., office and is an internationally known expert in the economics of the automotive and airlines industries. Prior to joining CRA, Dr. Eads was vice president and chief economist at General Motors Corporation. He frequently represented the corporation before congressional committees and federal regulatory agencies. He has served as a member of the President's Council of Economic Advisers and as a special assistant to the assistant attorney general in the Antitrust Division of the U.S. Department of Justice. Dr. Eads has published numerous books and articles on the impact of government on business and has taught at several major universities, including Harvard and Princeton.

★ Member, Subcommittee on Strategies and Models for Providing Health Insurance.

Jack Ebeler, M.P.A.,★ is president and chief executive officer of Alliance of Community Health Plans. Previously, he was the senior vice president and director of the Health Care Group of The Robert Wood Johnson Foundation, focusing on the goals of improving access to care and improving care for people with chronic conditions. He served as deputy assistant secretary for health policy and as acting assistant secretary for planning and evaluation for the U.S. Department of Health and Human Services (DHHS), where he led department-wide policy efforts on priority health initiatives. Before serving at DHHS, Jack was the vice president of Minnesota-based Group Health, Inc., now HealthPartners. He is on the Board of Directors of Families USA and the Health Care Services Board of the Institute of Medicine. Jack's undergraduate degree is from Dickinson College. He has a master's degree in public administration from Harvard University's John F. Kennedy School of Government.

Sandra R. Hernández, M.D., is chief executive officer of the San Francisco Foundation, a community foundation serving California's five Bay Area counties. It is one of the largest community foundations in the country. Dr. Hernández is a primary care internist who previously held a number of positions within the San Francisco Department of Public Health, including director of the AIDS Office, director of community public health, county health officer, and director of health for the City and County of San Francisco. She was appointed to and served on President Clinton's Advisory Commission on Consumer Protection and Quality in the Healthcare Industry. Among the many honors and awards bestowed on her, Dr. Hernández was named by *Modern Healthcare* magazine as one of the top ten health care leaders for the next century. Dr. Hernández is a graduate of Yale University, Tufts School of Medicine, and the John F. Kennedy School of Government at Harvard University. She is on the faculty of the University of California at San Francisco School of Medicine and maintains an active clinical practice at San Francisco General Hospital in the AIDS Clinic.

Willard G. Manning, Ph.D., is professor in the Department of Health Studies, Pritzker School of Medicine, and in the Harris School of Public Policy at The University of Chicago. His primary research focus has been the effects of health insurance and alternative delivery systems on the use of health services and health status. He is an expert in statistical issues in cost-effectiveness analysis and small area variations. His recent work has included examination of mental health services use and outcomes in a Medicaid population, and cost-effectiveness analysis of screening and treating depression in primary care. Dr. Manning is a member of the Institute of Medicine.

Barbara Matula, M.P.A.,★ has spent the past 20 years administering Medicaid, beginning with a position at the State Budget Office in North Carolina. In 1979 she was appointed the state's Medicaid director and held this position for 15 years. Presently, Ms. Matula is the Director of Health Care Programs at North Carolina

Medical Society Foundation. She works for the philanthropic arm of the society, which is dedicated to improving access to care for the poor, uninsured, and underserved in North Carolina and improving the ability of physicians to serve them. Ms. Matula helped to establish the National Academy for State Health Policy and has served as its chair since its founding in 1987. As a member of the National Infant Mortality Commission, she helped to author legislation that broke the welfare link to Medicaid eligibility. Ms. Matula received a National Public Service Award in 1995.

James J. Mongan, M.D., is president and chief executive officer of Partners HealthCare, Inc., and was previously president of Massachusetts General Hospital. Dr. Mongan served as assistant surgeon general in the U.S. Department of Health and Human Services; as former associate director for health and human resources, domestic policy staff, the White House; and as former deputy assistant secretary for health policy, U.S. Department of Health, Education and Welfare. Dr. Mongan is chair of the Task Force on the Future of Health Insurance for Working Americans, a nonpartisan effort of the Commonwealth Fund to address the implications of the changing U.S. workforce and economy for the availability and affordability of health insurance. He is also a member of the Kaiser Family Foundation Board and the Kaiser Commission on Medicaid and the Uninsured.

Len Nichols, Ph.D.,★ is vice president of the Center for Studying Health System Change. He is a health policy expert who has published extensively on a variety of topics, including insurance market regulation, the effect of tax policy on health insurance purchase decisions, and private insurance options for Medicare. He previously served as principal research associate at the Urban Institute, senior advisor for health policy at the U.S. Office of Management and Budget, and chair of the economics department at Wellesley College.

Christopher Queram, M.A.,★ has been chief executive officer of the Employer Health Care Alliance Cooperative (The Alliance) of Madison, Wisconsin, since 1993. The Alliance is a purchasing cooperative owned by more than 160 member companies that contracts with providers; manages and reports cost and utilization data; performs consumer education and advocacy; and designs employer and provider quality initiatives and reports. Prior to his current position, Mr. Queram served as vice president for programs at Meriter Hospital, a 475-bed hospital in Madison. Mr. Queram is a member of the board of The Leapfrog Group and serves as treasurer. He is also a member and past chair of the board of the National Business Coalition on Health. Mr. Queram was a member of the President's Advisory Commission on Consumer Protection and Quality in the Health Care Industry, served as a member of the Planning Committee for the National Quality Forum, and continues as chair of the Purchaser Council and board member of the Forum. He is a member of the Wisconsin Board on Health Information and the Board of the Wisconsin Private Employer Health Care Coverage program. He holds a master's degree in health services administration from the University of Wisconsin at Madison and is a fellow in the American College of Healthcare Executives.

Shoshanna Sofaer, Dr.P.H.$\star$† is the Robert P. Luciano Professor of Health Care Policy at the School of Public Affairs, Baruch College, in New York City. She completed her master's and doctoral degrees in public health at the University of California, Berkeley; taught for 6 years at the University of California, Los Angeles, School of Public Health; served on the faculty of George Washington University Medical Center, where she was professor, associate dean for research of the School of Public Health and Health Services, and director of the Center for Health Outcomes Improvement Research. Dr. Sofaer's research interests include providing information to individual consumers on the performance of the health care system; assessing the impact of information on both consumers and the system; developing consumer-relevant performance measures; and improving the responsiveness of the Medicare program to the needs of current and future cohorts of older persons and persons with disabilities. In addition, Dr. Sofaer studies the role of community coalitions in pursuing public health and health care system reform objectives and has extensive experience in the evaluation of community health improvement interventions. She has studied the determinants of health insurance status among the near-elderly, including early retirees. Dr. Sofaer served as co-chair of the Working Group on Coverage for Low Income and Non-Working Families for the White House Task Force on Health Care Reform in 1993 and co-chair of the Task Force on Medicare of the Century Foundation in New York City. She is a member of the Health Systems Study Section of the Agency for Healthcare Research and Quality.

Stephen J. Trejo, Ph.D., is associate professor in the Department of Economics at the University of Texas at Austin. His primary research focus has been in the field of labor economics. He has examined the response of labor market participants to the incentives created by market opportunities, government policies, and the institutional environment. Specific research topics include the economic effects of overtime pay regulation; immigrant labor market outcomes and welfare recipiency; the impact of labor unions on compensation, employment, and work schedules; the importance of sector-specific skills; and the relative economic status of Mexican Americans.

Reed V. Tuckson, M.D.,$\star$ is senior vice president of consumer health and medical care advancement at UnitedHealth Group. Formerly, he was senior vice president, professional standards, at the American Medical Association. Dr.

---

†Chair, Subcommittee on Strategies and Models for Providing Health Insurance.

Tuckson was president of Charles R. Drew University School of Medicine and Science from 1991 to 1997. From 1986 to 1990, he was commissioner of public health for the District of Columbia. Dr. Tuckson serves on a number of health care, academic, and federal boards and committees and is a nationally known lecturer on topics concerning community-based medicine, the moral responsibilities of health professionals, and physician leadership. He currently serves on the IOM Roundtable on Research and Development of Drugs, Biologics, and Medical Devices and is a member of the Institute of Medicine.

Edward H. Wagner, M.D., M.P.H., F.A.C.P.,⋆ is a general internist–epidemiologist and director of the W.A. (Sandy) MacColl Institute for Healthcare Innovation at the Center for Health Studies, Group Health Cooperative. He is also professor of health services at the University of Washington School of Public Health and Community Medicine. Current research interests include the development and testing of population-based care models for diabetes, frail elderly, and other chronic illnesses; the evaluation of the health and cost impacts of chronic disease and cancer interventions; and interventions to prevent disability and reduce depressive symptoms in older adults. Dr. Wagner has written 2 books and more than 200 journal articles. He serves on the editorial boards of *Health Services Research* and the *Journal of Clinical Epidemiology* and acts as a consultant to multiple federal agencies and private foundations. He recently served as senior advisor on managed care initiatives in the Director's Office of the National Institutes of Health. Dr. Wagner directs Improving Chronic Illness Care (ICIC), a national program of The Robert Wood Johnson Foundation. The overall goal of ICIC is to assist health systems in improving their care of chronic illness through quality improvement and evaluation, research, and dissemination. Dr. Wagner is also principal investigator of the Cancer Research Network, a National Cancer Institute-funded consortium of 10 health maintenance organizations conducting collaborative cancer effectiveness research.

Lawrence Wallack, Dr.P.H., is professor of public health and director, School of Community Health, at Portland State University. He is also professor of public health, University of California, Berkeley. Dr. Wallack's primary interest is in the role of mass communications, particularly the news media, in shaping public health issues. His current research is on how public health issues are framed in print and broadcast news. He is principal author of *Media Advocacy and Public Health: Power for Prevention* and *News for a Change: An Advocate's Guide to Working with the Media*. He is also co-editor of *Mass Communications and Public Health: Complexities and Conflicts*. Dr. Wallack has published extensively on topics related to prevention, health promotion, and community interventions. Specific content areas of his research and intervention work have included alcohol, tobacco, violence, handguns, sexually transmitted diseases, cervical and breast cancer, affirmative action, suicide, and childhood lead poisoning. Dr. Wallack was a member of the IOM Committee on Communication for Behavior Change in the 21st Century: Improving the Health of Diverse Populations.

Alan Weil, J.D., M.P.P.,★ directs the Assessing the New Federalism project at the Urban Institute. This project, the largest in the Institute's 34-year history, monitors, describes, and assesses the effects of changes in federal and state health, welfare, and social services programs. Mr. Weil was formerly executive director of the Colorado Department of Health Care Policy and Financing—the cabinet position responsible for Colorado's Medicaid and Medically Indigent programs, health data collection and analysis functions, health policy development, and health care reform. He was also health policy adviser to Colorado Governor Roy Romer, program director of the Colorado Children's Campaign, and legal counsel to the Massachusetts Department of Medical Security. He holds a bachelor's degree in economics and political science from the University of California at Berkeley, a master of public policy degree from the John F. Kennedy School of Government at Harvard, and a J.D. from Harvard Law School.

Institute of Medicine Staff

Wilhelmine Miller, M.S., Ph.D., is a senior program officer in the Division of Health Care Services. She served as staff to the Committee on Immunization Finance Policy and Practices, conducting and directing case studies of health care financing and public health services. Prior to joining the Institute of Medicine, Dr. Miller was an adjunct faculty member in the Departments of Philosophy at Georgetown University and Trinity College, teaching political philosophy, ethics, and public policy. She received her doctorate from Georgetown, with studies and research in bioethics and issues of social justice. In 1994–1995, Dr. Miller was a consultant to the President's Advisory Committee on Human Radiation Experiments. Dr. Miller was a program analyst in the U.S. Department of Health and Human Services for 14 years, responsible for policy development and regulatory review in areas including hospital and health maintenance organization payment, prescription drug benefits, and child health. Her M.S. from Harvard University is in health policy and management.

Dianne Miller Wolman, M.G.A., joined the Health Care Services Division of the Institute of Medicine in 1999 as a senior program officer. She directed the study that resulted in the IOM report *Medicare Laboratory Payment Policy: Now and in the Future*, released in 2000. Her previous work experience in the health field has been varied and extensive, focused on finance and reimbursement in insurance programs. She came to the IOM from the U.S. General Accounting Office, where she was a senior evaluator on studies of the Health Care Financing Administration, its management capacity, and its oversight of Medicare contractors. Prior to that, she was a reimbursement policy specialist at a national association representing nonprofit providers of long-term care services. Her earlier positions included policy analysis and management in the Office of the Secretary of the U.S. Department of Health and Human Services and work with a peer review organization, a governor's task force on access to health care, and a third-party administrator for very large health plans. In addition, she was policy director for a state Medicaid rate-setting commission. She has a bachelor's degree in sociology from Brandeis University and a master's degree in government administration from Wharton Graduate School, University of Pennsylvania.

Lynne Page Snyder, Ph.D., M.P.H., is a program officer in the IOM Division of Health Care Services. She came to the IOM from the U.S. Department of Health and Human Services, where she worked as a public historian, documenting and writing about past federal activities in medicine, health care, and public health. In addition, she has worked for the Social Science Research Council's Committee on the Urban Underclass and served as a graduate fellow at the Smithsonian Institution's National Museum of American History. She has published on 20th-century health policy, occupational and environmental health, and minority health. Current research interests include health literacy and access to care by low-income seniors. She earned her doctorate in the history and sociology of science from the University of Pennsylvania (1994), working under Rosemary Stevens, and received her M.P.H. from the Johns Hopkins School of Hygiene and Public Health (2000).

Tracy McKay, B.A.,† is a research associate in the IOM Division of Health Care Services. She has worked on several projects, including the National Roundtable on Health Care Quality; Children, Health Insurance, and Access to Care; Quality of Health Care in America; and a study on non-heart-beating organ donors. She has assisted in the research for the National Quality Report on Health Care Delivery, Immunization Finance Policies and Practices, and Extending Medicare Coverage for Preventive and Other Services, and helped develop this project on the consequences of uninsurance from its inception. Ms. McKay received her B.A. in sociology from Vassar College in 1996.

Ryan L. Palugod, B.S., is a senior program assistant in the IOM Division of Health Care Services. He has worked on several projects, including the Immunization Finance Dissemination, and Evaluation of Vaccine Purchase Financing in the United States. Prior to joining the project staff in 2001, he worked as an administrative assistant with the American Association of Homes, Services for the Aging. He graduated with honors from Towson University in 1999 with a degree in health care management.

---

†Served until August, 2003.

References

Achman, Lori, and Deborah Chollet. 2001. *Insuring the Uninsurable: An Overview of State High-Risk Health Insurance Pools*. Pub. No. 472. New York: The Commonwealth Fund.

Adcox, Seanna. 2002. Advocates Say Easy Health Access Works. Large Number of Enrollees for Temporary Program Called Sign of Need to Cut Red Tape. *Albany Times-Union*. January 21, 2002.

Agency for Healthcare Research and Quality (AHRQ). 2001. *Health Care Expenses in the United States, 1996*. Washington, DC: Agency for Healthcare Research and Quality.

Alteras, Tanya T. 2001. *Understanding the Dynamics of Crowding Out: Defining Public/Private Coverage Substitution for Policy and Research*. Accessed June 19, 2001. Available at: http://www.hcfo.net.

Anderson, Gerard F., Varduhi Petrosyan, and Peter Hussey. 2002. *Multinational Comparisons of Health Systems Data, 2002*. New York: The Commonwealth Fund.

Anderson, Gerard F., Uwe E. Reinhardt, Peter S. Hussey, and Varduhi Petrosyan. 2003. It's the Prices, Stupid: Why the United States Is So Different from Other Countries. *Health Affairs* 22(3):89-105.

Aron, David C., Howard S. Gordon, David L. DiGiuseppe, Dwain L. Harper, et al. 2000. Variations in Risk-Adjusted Cesarean Delivery Rates According to Race and Health Insurance. *Medical Care* 38(1):35-44.

Associated Press. 2001. *Arizona Lawmakers Approve Bill to Cover Dialysis, Chemotherapy for Undocumented Immigrants*. Accessed December 21, 2001. Available at: http://www.kaisernetwork.org/daily_reports/print_report.cfm?DR_ID=8712&dr_cat=3.

———. 2003. Maine Senate to Vote on Health Plan. *New York Times*. June 13, 2003.

Ayanian, John Z., Betsy A. Kohler, Toshi Abe, and Arnold M. Epstein. 1993. The Relation Between Health Insurance Coverage and Clinical Outcomes Among Women with Breast Cancer. *New England Journal of Medicine* 329(5):326-331.

Ayanian, John Z., Joel S. Weissman, Eric C. Schneider, Jack A. Ginsburg, and Alan M. Zaslavsky. 2000. Unmet Health Needs of Uninsured Adults in the United States. *Journal of the American Medical Association* 284(16):2061-2069.

Baker, David W., Joseph J. Sudano, Jeffrey M. Albert, Elaine A. Borawski, et al. 2001. Lack of Health Insurance and Decline in Overall Health in Late Middle Age. *New England Journal of Medicine* 345(15):1106-1112.

Baldwin, Laura-Mae, Eric H. Larson, Frederick A. Connell, Daniel Nordlund, et al. 1998. The Effect of Expanding Medicaid Prenatal Services on Birth Outcomes. *American Journal of Public Health* 88(11):1623-1629.

Beauchamp, Dan E., and Ronald L. Rouse. 1990. Universal New York Health Care: A Single-Payer Strategy Linking Cost Control and Universal Access. *New England Journal of Medicine* 323(10): 640-644.

Beckles, Gloria L. A., Michael M. Engelgau, K. M. V. Narayan, William H. Herman, et al. 1998. Population-Based Assessment of the Level of Care Among Adults with Diabetes in the U.S. *Diabetes Care* 21(9):1432-1438.

Berk, Marc L., and Alan C. Monheit. 2001. The Concentration of Health Care Expenditures, Revisited. *Health Affairs* 20(2):9-18.

Bernstein, Amy B. 1999. *Insurance Status and Use of Health Services by Pregnant Women.* Washington, DC: March of Dimes.

Bhandari, Shailesh, and Robert Mills. 2003. *Dynamics of Economic Well-Being: Health Insurance 1996-1999.* Current Population Reports. P70-92. Washington, DC: U.S. Census Bureau.

Birnbaum, Michael. 2000. *Expanding Coverage to Parents Through Medicaid Section 1931.* Washington, DC: Academy for Health Services Research and Health Policy, State Coverage Initiatives.

Blue Cross Blue Shield Association. 2000. *State Legislative Health Care and Insurance Issues: 2000 Survey of Plans.* Washington, DC: Blue Cross Blue Shield Association.

Blumberg, Linda J. 2001. *Health Insurance Tax Credits: Potential for Expanding Coverage.* Health Policy Briefs. Washington, DC: The Urban Institute.

Bovbjerg, Randall, Charles C. Griffin, and Caitlin E. Carroll. 1993. U.S. Health Care Coverage and Costs: Historical Development and Choices for the 1990s. *Journal of Law, Medicine, and Ethics* 21(2):141-162.

Bovbjerg, Randall R., and Frank C. Ullman. 2002. *Recent Changes in Health Policy for Low-Income People in Massachusetts.* State Update No. 17. Washington, DC: The Urban Institute.

Boyd, Donald J. 2003. Health Care Within the Larger State Budget. Pp. 59-110 in: *Federalism and Health Policy,* John Holahan, Alan Weil, and Joshua Wiener, eds. Washington, DC: The Urban Institute.

Braveman, Paula, Susan Egerter, Trude Bennett, and Jonathan Showstack. 1991. Differences in Hospital Resource Allocation Among Sick Newborns According to Insurance Coverage. *Journal of the American Medical Association* 266(23):3300-3308.

Breen, Nancy, Diane Wagener, Martin L. Brown, William Davis, et al. 2001. Progress in Cancer Screening over a Decade. Results of Cancer Screening from the 1987, 1992 and 1998 National Health Interview Surveys. *Journal of the National Cancer Institute* 93(22):1704-1713.

Broaddus, Matthew, and Leighton Ku. 2000. *Nearly 95 Percent of Low-Income Uninsured Children Now Are Eligible for Medicaid or SCHIP.* Washington, DC: Center on Budget and Policy Priorities.

Broaddus, Matthew, Shannon Blaney, Annie Dude, Jocelyn Guyer, et al. 2002. *Expanding Family Coverage: States' Medicaid Eligibility Policies for Working Families in the Year 2000.* Washington, DC: Center on Budget and Policy Priorities.

Brown, E. R., Ninez Ponce, Thomas Rice, and Shana Alex Lavarreda. 2002. *The State of Health Insurance in California: Findings From the 2001 California Health Interview Survey.* Los Angeles: UCLA Center for Health Policy Research.

Brown, Lawrence D., and Michael S. Sparer. 2001. Window Shopping: State Health Reform Politics in the 1990s. *Health Affairs* 20(1):50-67.

Bundorf, M. Kate, and Mark V. Pauly. 2002. *Is Health Insurance Affordable for the Uninsured?* Working Paper No.9281. Cambridge, MA: National Bureau of Economic Research.

Burstin, Helen R., Stuart R. Lipsitz, and Troyen A. Brennan. 1992. Socioeconomic Status and Risk for Substandard Medical Care. *Journal of the American Medical Association* 268(17):2383-2387.

Burstin, Helen R., Katherine Swartz, Anne C. O'Neill, E. John Orav, et al. 1998. The Effect of Change of Health Insurance on Access to Care. *Inquiry* 35:389-397.

Butler, Patricia. 2000. *ERISA Pre-Emption Manual for State Health Policy Makers.* Washington, DC: Academy for Health Services Research and Health Policy, State Coverage Initiatives.

―――. 2002. *Revisiting Pay or Play: How States Could Expand Employer-Based Coverage Within ERISA Constraints.* Portland, ME: National Academy for State Health Policy.

Butler, Stuart M. 2001. Reforming the Tax Treatment of Health Care to Achieve Universal Coverage. Pp. 23-42 in: *Covering America: Real Remedies for the Uninsured,* Jack A. Meyer and Elliot K. Wicks, eds. Washington, DC: Economic and Social Research Institute.

Carlisle, David M., Barbara D. Leake, and Martin F. Shapiro. 1997. Racial and Ethnic Disparities in the Use of Cardiovascular Procedures: Associations with Type of Health Insurance. *American Journal of Public Health* 87(2):263-267.

Carpenter, Charles C. J., Margaret A. Fischl, Scott M. Hammer, Martin S. Hirsch, et al. 1996. Antiretroviral Therapy for HIV Infection in 1996. *Journal of the American Medical Association* 276(2):146-154.

―――. 1998. Antiretroviral Therapy for HIV Infection in 1998: Updated Recommendations of the International AIDS Society-USA Panel. *Journal of the American Medical Association* 280(1):78-86.

Carrier, Paul. 2003. Health-Care Bill Close to Passage in Legislature. *Portland Press Herald.* June 13, 2003.

Catholic Health Association. 2002. *A Commitment to Caring. The Role of Catholic Hospitals in the Health Care Safety Net.* Accessed November 18, 2002. Available at: http://chausa.org/PUBLICPO/SAFETYNET.ASP.

Centers for Disease Control and Prevention. 2002. *Infant Mortality Rates, Fetal Mortality Rates, and Perinatal Rates, According to Race: United States, Selected Years 1950-99.* Table 23. Accessed July 7, 2003. Available at: http://www.cdc.gov/nchs/data/hus/tables/2002/02hus023.pdf.

―――. 2003. *Early Release of Selected Estimates Based on Data from the 2002 National Health Interview Survey.* Accessed October 1, 2003. Available at: http://www.cdc.gov/nchs/data/nhis/earlyrelease/200306_01.pdf.

Centers for Medicare and Medicaid Services (CMS). 2003a. *Fiscal Year 2002 Number of Children Ever Enrolled in SCHIP—Preliminary Data Summary.* Accessed April 2, 2003. Available at: http://www.cms.gov/schip/schip02.pdf.

―――. 2003b. *State Children's Health Insurance Program Plan Activity Map.* Accessed April 2, 2003. Available at: http://www.cms.gov/schip/chip-map.asp.

Chernew, Michael, David Cutler, and Patricia Seliger Keenan. 2002. *Rising Health Care Costs and the Decline in Insurance Coverage.* Ann Arbor, MI: Economic Research Initiative on the Uninsured.

Child Health Insurance Initiative. 2002. *SCHIP Disenrollment and State Policies.* Washington, DC: Agency for Healthcare Research and Quality.

Chollet, Deborah, and Lori Achman. 2003. *Approaching Universal Coverage: Minnesota's Health Insurance Programs.* Pub. No. 566. New York: The Commonwealth Fund.

Chollet, Deborah, and Adele Kirk. 1998. *Understanding Individual Health Insurance Markets: Structure, Practices, and Products in Ten States.* Menlo Park, CA: The Henry J. Kaiser Family Foundation.

Chollet, Deborah, Glen Mays, January Angeles, Roland McDevitt, et al. 2002. *Feasibility of a Single-Payer Health Plan Model for the State of Maine.* MPR Reference No. 8889-300. Washington, DC: Mathematica Policy Research.

Collins, Sara R., Cathy Schoen, and Katie Tenney. 2003. *Rites of Passage? Why Young Adults Become Uninsured and How New Policies Can Help.* Issue Brief No. 649. New York: The Commonwealth Fund.

Commonwealth Fund. 2001. *A Shared Responsibility: Academic Health Centers and the Provision of Care to the Poor and Uninsured.* New York: The Commonwealth Fund, Task Force on Academic Health Centers. ·

Congressional Budget Office (CBO). 2002. *Glossary of Budgetary and Economic Terms.* Accessed November 25, 2002. Available at: http://www.cbo.gov/showdoc.cfm?index=3280&sequence=0.

―――. 2003. *How Many People Lack Health Insurance and for How Long?* Washington, DC: Congress of the United States and Congressional Budget Office.

Congressional Quarterly. 1973. *Congress and the Nation: A Review of Government and Politics.* Vol. 3 (1969-1972). Washington, DC: Congressional Quarterly Service.

———. 1977. *Congress and the Nation: A Review of Government and Politics.* Vol. 4 (1973-1976). Washington, DC: Congressional Quarterly Service.

Conover, Christopher J., and Hester H. Davies. 2000. *The Role of TennCare in Health Policy for Low-Income People in Tennessee.* Occasional Paper No. 33. Washington, DC: The Urban Institute.

Conviser, Richard. N.d. *A Brief History of the Oregon Health Plan and its Features.* Portland, OR: State of Oregon.

Cooper, Philip F., and Barbara S. Schone. 1997. More Offers, Fewer Takers for Employer-Based Health Insurance: 1987 and 1996. *Health Affairs* 16(6):142-149.

Cooper-Patrick, Lisa, Rosa M. Crum, Laura A. Pratt, William W. Eaton, et al. 1999. The Psychiatric Profile of Patients with Chronic Disease Who Do Not Receive Regular Medical Care. *International Journal of Psychiatry* 29(2):165-180.

Corrigan, Janet M., Ann Greiner, and Shari M. Erickson (eds.). 2003. *Fostering Rapid Advances in Health Care.* Washington, DC: The National Academies Press.

Cummings, Doyle M., Lauren Whetstone, Amy Shende, and David Weismiller. 2000. Predictors of Screenings Mammography: Implications for Office Practice. *Archives of Family Medicine* 9(9):870-875.

Cunningham, Peter. 2003. *Personal communication with IOM staff.* Washington, DC: Center for Studying Health System Change.

Cunningham, Peter, and Ha T. Tu. 1997. A Changing Picture of Uncompensated Care. *Health Affairs* 14(4):167-175.

Cunningham, Peter J., Jack Hadley, and James D Reschovsky. 2002. *The Effects of SCHIP on Children's Health Insurance Coverage.* Accessed April 7, 2003. Available at: http://www.hschange.com/CONTENT/510.

Cunningham, Robert, III, and Cunningham, Robert M. Jr. 1997. *The Blues. A History of the Blue Cross and Blue Shield System.* DeKalb, IL: Northern Illinois University Press.

Currie, Janet, and Jonathan Gruber. 1996a. Health Insurance Eligibility, Utilization of Medical Care, and Child Health. *The Quarterly Journal of Economics* 111(2):431-466.

———. 1996b. Saving Babies: The Efficacy and Cost of Recent Changes in the Medicaid Eligibility of Pregnant Women. *Journal of Political Economy* 104(6):1263-1296.

Curtis, Richard E., and Edward Neuschler. 2002. *Tax Credits for Individual Health Insurance: Effects on Employer Coverage and Refinements to Improve Overall Coverage Rates.* Washington, DC: Economic and Social Research Institute.

Curtis, Richard E., Edward Neuschler, and Rafe Forland. 2001. Consumer-Choice Purchasing Pools: Past Tense, Future Perfect? *Health Affairs* 20(1):164-168.

Custer, William S., and Pat Ketsche. 2000. *Employment-Based Health Insurance Coverage.* Washington, DC: Health Insurance Association of America.

Cutler, David M. 2002. *Employee Costs and the Decline in Health Insurance Coverage.* Boston, MA: Harvard University and National Bureau of Economic Research.

Cutler, David M., and Jonathan Gruber. 1996a. Does Public Insurance Crowd Out Private Insurance? *Quarterly Journal of Economics* 111:391-430.

———. 1996b. The Effect of Medicaid Expansions on Public Insurance, Private Insurance, and Redistribution. *The American Economic Review* 86(2):378-383.

———. 1997. Medicaid and Private Insurance: Evidence and Implications. *Health Affairs* 16(1):194-200.

Cutler, David M., and Elizabeth Richardson. 1997. Measuring the Health of the United States Population. *Brookings Papers on Economic Activity. Microeconomics:*217-271.

Dafny, Leemore, and Jonathan Gruber. 2000. *Does Public Insurance Improve the Efficiency of Medical Care? Medicaid Expansions and Child Hospitalizations.* Cambridge, MA: National Bureau of Economic Research.

Daumit, Gail, Judith A. Hermann, Josef Coresh, and Neil R. Powe. 1999. Use of Cardiovascular Procedures Among Black Persons and White Persons: A 7-Year Nationwide Study in Patients with Renal Disease. *Annals of Internal Medicine* 130(3):173-182.

Daumit, Gail L., Judith A. Hermann, and Neil R. Powe. 2000. Relation of Gender and Health Insurance to Cardiovascular Procedure Use in Persons with Progression of Chronic Renal Disease. *Medical Care* 38(4):354-365.

Davis, Karen. 2001. Universal Coverage in the United States: Lessons from Experience of the 20th Century. *Journal of Urban Health* 78(1):46-58.

Davis, Karen, and Cathy Schoen. 2003. *Creating Consensus on Coverage Choices.* Accessed May 1, 2003. Available at: http://www.healthaffairs.org/WebExclusives/Davis_Web_Excl_042303.htm.

Davis, Karen, Cathy Schoen, and Stephen C. Schoenbaum. 2000. A 2020 Vision for American Health Care. *Archives of Internal Medicine* 160(22):3357-3362.

Derickson, Alan. 2002. Health for Three-Thirds of the Nation. *American Journal of Public Health* 92(2):180-190.

Dick, Andrew W. 1994. Will Employer Mandates Really Work? Another Look at Hawaii. *Health Affairs* 13(1):343-349.

Docteur, Elizabeth, Hannes Suppanz, and Jaejoon Woo. 2003. *The US Health System: An Assessment and Prospective Directions for Reform. Economics Department Working Papers No. 350.* Accessed April 17, 2003. Available at: http://www.oecd.org/eco.

Dorn, Stan. 2003. *The Trade Act of 2002: Coverage Options for States.* In Focus. Washington, DC: AcademyHealth, State Coverage Initiatives.

Doty, Michelle, and Cathy Schoen. 2001. *Maintaining Health Insurance During a Recession: Likely COBRA Eligibility.* Issue Brief No. 513. New York: The Commonwealth Fund.

Doyle, James. 2003. *As Medicaid Enrollment Has Surged, Composition of Caseload Has Changed.* Background Paper. Accessed July 7, 2003. Available at: http://www.ibo.nyc.ny.us.

Doyle, Joseph J. 2001. *Does Health Insurance Affect Treatment Decisions & Patient Outcomes? Using Automobile Accidents As Unexpected Health Shocks.* Chicago: University of Chicago, Unpublished MS.

Draper, Debra A., Linda R. Brewster, Lawrence D. Brown, Lance Heineccius, et al. 2001a. *Financial Pressures Continue to Plague Hospitals: Northern New Jersey.* Washington, DC: Center for Studying Health System Change.

Draper, Debra A., Linda R. Brewster, Lawrence D. Brown, Carolyn A. Watts, et al. 2001b. *Rapid Population Growth Attracts National Firm: Phoenix, Arizona.* Community Report, Third Visit, 2000-2001. Washington, DC: Center for Studying Health System Change.

Dubay, Lisa. 1999. *Expansions in Public Health Insurance and Crowd Out: What the Evidence Says.* Accessed July 2, 2001. Available at: http://www.kff.org.

Dubay, Lisa, Jennifer Haley, and Genevieve Kenney. 2002a. *Children's Eligibility for Medicaid and SCHIP: A View From 2000.* Series B, No. B-41.Washington, DC: The Urban Institute.

Dubay, Lisa, Ian Hill, and Genevieve Kenney. 2002b. *Five Things Everyone Should Know About SCHIP.* Series B, No. 40. Washington, DC: The Urban Institute.

Dubay, Lisa, Genevieve Kenney, and Jennifer Haley. 2002c. *Children's Participation in Medicaid and SCHIP: Early in the SCHIP Era.* Series B, No. B-40. Washington, DC: The Urban Institute.

Duchon, Lisa, Cathy Schoen, Michelle M. Doty, Karen Davis, et al. 2001. *Security Matters: How Instability in Health Insurance Puts U.S. Workers at Risk: Findings from the 2001 Health Insurance Survey.* Pub. 512. New York: The Commonwealth Fund.

Eastman, A. B., Charles L. Rice, David G. Bishop, and J. David Richardson. 1991. An Analysis of the Critical Problem of Trauma Center Reimbursement. *Journal of Trauma* 31(7):920-925.

Edmunds, Margo, and Molly Joel Coye (eds.). 1998. *America's Children: Health Insurance and Access to Care.* Washington, DC: National Academy Press.

Etheredge, Lynn. 1990. Universal Health Insurance: Lessons of the 1970s, Prospects for the 1990s. *Frontiers of Health Services Management* 6(4):3-50.

Etheredge, Lynn, and Stan Dorn. 2003. *Health Insurance for Laid-Off Workers: A Time for Action.* Current Policy Series No. 5. Washington, DC: Economic and Social Research Institute.

Fairbrother, Gerry, Heidi Park, and Michael Gusmano. 2002. How Community Health Centers Are Coping with Their Uninsured Caseloads. *National Association of Community Health Centers 27th Policy and Issues Forum* (Washington, DC). New York: The Commonwealth Fund.

Faulkner, Lisa A., and Helen H. Schauffler. 1997. The Effect of Health Insurance Coverage on the Appropriate Use of Recommended Clinical Preventive Services. *American Journal of Preventive Medicine* 13(6):453-458.

Feder, Judith, Larry Levitt, Ellen O'Brien, and Diane Rowland. 2001. Assessing the Combination of Public Programs and Tax Credits. Pp. 45-56 in: *Covering America: Real Remedies for the Uninsured,* Jack A. Meyer and Elliot K. Wicks, eds. Washington, DC: Economic and Social Research Institute.

Felland, Laurie, and Andrea M. Benoit. 2001. *Communities Play Key Role in Extending Public Health Insurance to Children.* Issue Brief No. 44. Washington, DC: Center for Studying Health System Change.

Felt-Lisk, Suzanne, Megan McHugh, and Embry Howell. 2001. *Study of Safety Net Provider Capacity to Care for Low-Income Uninsured Patients. Final Report.* Washington, DC: Mathematica Policy Research.

Field, Marilyn J., Kathleen N. Lohr, and Karl D. Yordy (eds.). 1993. *Assessing Health Care Reform.* Washington, DC: National Academy Press.

Fish-Parcham, Cheryl. 2001. *Getting Less Care: The Uninsured with Chronic Health Conditions.* Washington, DC: Families USA Foundation.

Fossett, James W., and Courtney E. Burke. 2003. *Managing Medicaid Take-Up: Is Medicaid Retrenching? State Budgets and Medicaid Enrollment in 2002.* New York: The Nelson A. Rockefeller Institute of Government.

Fox, Daniel M. 1986. *Health Policies, Health Politics: The Experience of Britain and America, 1911-1965.* Princeton, NJ: Princeton University Press.

Fox, Daniel M., and Daniel C. Schaffer. 1989. Health Policy and ERISA: Interest Groups and Semipreemption. *Journal of Health Politics, Policy, and Law* 14(2):239-260.

Franks, Peter, Carolyn M. Clancy, and Marthe R. Gold. 1993a. Health Insurance and Mortality: Evidence from a National Cohort. *Journal of the American Medical Association* 270(6):737-741.

Franks, Peter, Carolyn M. Clancy, Marthe R. Gold, et al. 1993b. Health Insurance and Subjective Health Status: Data from the 1987 National Medical Expenditure Survey. *American Journal of Public Health* 83(9):1295-1299.

Freudenheim, Milt. 2003. Many California Employers Face Health Care Mandate. *New York Times.* September 17, 2003.

Fronstin, Paul. 2000. *Sources of Health Insurance and Characteristics of the Uninsured: Analysis of the March 2000 Current Population Survey.* Washington, DC: Employee Benefit Research Institute.

———. 2002. *Sources of Health Insurance: Analysis of the March 2002 Current Population Survey.* EBRI Issue Brief No. 252. Washington, DC: Employee Benefit Research Institute.

Gabel, Jon. 1999. Job-Based Health Insurance, 1977-1998: The Accidental System Under Scrutiny. *Health Affairs* 18(6):62-74.

Gabel, Jon R., Kelley Dhont, and Jeremy Pickreign. 2002. *Are Tax Credits Alone the Solution to Affordable Health Insurance?* Pub. No. 527. New York: The Commonwealth Fund.

Gaskin, Darrell J. 1999. *Safety Net Hospitals: Essential Providers of Public Health and Specialty Services.* New York: The Commonwealth Fund.

Gaskin, Darrell J., and Jack Needleman. 2003. The Impact of Uninsured Populations on the Availability of Hospital Services and Financial Status in Hospital Urban Areas. Pp. 205-220 in: *A Shared Destiny: Community Effects of Uninsurance,* Institute of Medicine. Washington, DC: The National Academies Press.

Glied, Sherry. 2003. Health Care Costs: On the Rise Again. *Journal of Economic Perspectives* 17(2):125-148.

Gold, Marsha R., Jessica Mittler, Anna Aizer, Barbara Lyons, et al. 2001. Health Insurance Expansion Through States in a Pluralistic System. *Journal of Health Politics, Policy and Law* 26(3):581-615.

Goldman, Dana P., Jayanta Bhattcharya, Daniel F. McCaffrey, Naihua Duan, et al. 2001. Effect of Insurance on Mortality in an HIV-Positive Population in Care. *Journal of the American Statistical Association* 96(455):883-894.

Gribben, August. 2002. Hospitals Feel Pain of Mexico Crossings. *Washington Times.* Accessed March 18, 2002. Available at: http://www.washtimes.com/national/20020318-97583307.htm.

Gruber, Jonathan. 2001. A Private/Public Partnership for National Health Insurance. Pp. 59-71 in: *Covering America: Real Remedies for the Uninsured,* Jack A. Meyer and Elliot K. Wicks, eds. Washington, DC: Economic and Social Research Institute.

Gruber, Jonathan, and Maria Hanratty. 1995. The Labor-Market Effect of Introducing National Health Insurance: Evidence from Canada. *Journal of Business and Economic Statistics* 13(2):163-173.

Gusmano, Michael K., Gerry Fairbrother, and Heidi Park. 2002. Exploring the Limits of the Safety Net: Community Health Centers and Care for the Uninsured. *Health Affairs* 21(6):188-194.

Guyer, Jocelyn. 2003. *Medicaid and State Budgets: An Overview of Five States' Experiences in 2001.* Washington, DC: The Kaiser Commission on Medicaid and the Uninsured.

Haas, Jennifer S., Steven Udvarhelyi, and Arnold M. Epstein. 1993. The Effect of Health Coverage for Uninsured Pregnant Women on Maternal Health and the Use of Cesarean Section. *Journal of the American Medical Association* 270(1):61-64.

Hacker, Jacob. 1997. *The Road to Nowhere: The Genesis of President Clinton's Plan for Health Security.* Princeton, NY: Princeton University Press.

———. 2001. Medicare Plus: Increasing Health Coverage by Expanding Medicare. Pp. 75-100 in *Covering America: Real Remedies for the Uninsured.* Jack A. Meyer and Elliot K. Wicks, eds. Washington, DC: Economic and Social Research Institute.

Hadley, Jack. 2002. *Sicker and Poorer: The Consequences of Being Uninsured.* Washington, DC: The Henry J. Kaiser Family Foundation.

Hadley, Jack, and John Holahan. 2003a. Estimates of the Cost of Covering the Uninsured. *Health Affairs* Web Exclusive 22(4):W3-250-W3-265.

———. 2003b. How Much Medical Care Do the Uninsured Use and Who Pays for It? *Health Affairs* Web Exclusive (1):W66-W81.

Hadley, Jack, and James D. Reschovsky. 2002. *Tax Credits and the Affordability of Individual Health Insurance.* Washington, DC: Center for Studying Health System Change.

Haley, Jennifer M., and Stephen Zuckerman. 2000. *Health Insurance, Access, and Use: United States. Tabulations from the 1997 National Survey of America's Families.* Washington, DC: The Urban Institute.

———. 2003. *Is Lack of Coverage a Short- or Long-Term Condition?* Pub. No. 4122. Washington, DC: The Kaiser Commission on Medicaid and the Uninsured.

Hargraves, J. L., and Jack Hadley. 2003. The Contribution of Insurance Coverage and Community Resources to Reducing Racial/Ethnic Disparities in Access of Care. *Health Services Research* 38(3):809-829.

Haskell, Meg. 2003. Governor Announces Health Plan. Public-Private Entity to Rely on Surcharges. *Bangor News.* May 6, 2003.

The Hawaii Uninsured Project Leadership Group. 2002. *A Plan for Action: Striving to Make Health Care Available for All People in Hawaii.* Honolulu, HI: The Hawaii Uninsured Project.

Hawkins, Daniel R., and Sara Rosenbaum. 1998. The Challenges Facing Health Centers in a Changing Healthcare System. Pp. 99-122 in: *The Future U.S. Healthcare System: Who Will Care for the Poor and Uninsured?* Stuart H. Altman, Uwe E. Reinhardt, and Alexandra E. Shields, eds. Chicago: Health Administration Press.

Healthcare Leadership Council. 2003. *Trade Adjustment Assistance Act (TAA). Health Coverage Tax Credit (HCTC).* Washington, DC: Healthcare Leadership Council.

Heffler, Stephen, Sheila Smith, Sean Keehan, M. K. Clemens, et al. 2003. Health Spending Projections for 2002-2012. *Health Affairs* 22(2):W3-54-W3-65.

Heidenreich, Paul, and Mark McClellan. 2003. Biomedical Research and Then Some: The Causes of Technological Change in Heart Attack Treatment. In: *Measuring Gains from Medical Research: An Economic Approach.* Kevin Murphy and Robert H. Topel, eds. Chicago: University of Chicago Press.

Hillsborough County. 2003. *Health and Social Services-Hillsborough County Government Online.* Accessed April 11, 2003. Available at: http://www.hillsboroughcounty.org/health_ss/home.html.

Himmelstein, David U., and Steffie Woolhandler. 2003. National Health Insurance or Incremental Reform: Aim High, or At Our Feet? *American Journal of Public Health* 93(1):102-105.

Hoffman, Beatrix. 2001. *The Wages of Sickness: The Politics of Health Insurance in Progressive America.* Chapel Hill: University of North Carolina Press.

Hoffman, Catherine, and Alan Schlobohm. 2000. *Uninsured in America: A Chart Book.* 2nd ed. Washington, DC: The Henry J. Kaiser Family Foundation.

Hoffman, Catherine, and Marie Wang. 2003. *Health Insurance Coverage in America: 2001 Data Update.* Washington, DC: The Kaiser Commission on Medicaid and the Uninsured.

Hoffman, Catherine, Cathy Schoen, Diane Rowland, and Karen Davis. 2001. Gaps in Health Coverage Among Working-Age Americans and the Consequences. *Journal of Health Care for the Poor and Underserved* 12(3):273-289.

Holahan, John. 2002. *Variations Among States in Health Insurance Coverage and Medical Expenditures: How Much Is Too Much?* Washington, DC: The Urban Institute.

Holahan, John, and Johnny Kim. 2000. Why Does the Number of Uninsured Americans Continue to Grow? *Health Affairs* 19(4):188-196.

Holahan, John, and Mary Pohl. 2003. Leaders and Laggards in State Coverage Expansions. Pp. 179-214 in *Federalism and Health Policy*, John Holahan, Alan Weil, and Joshua M. Wiener, eds. Washington, DC: The Urban Institute.

Holahan, John, and Brenda Spillman. 2002. *Health Care Access for Uninsured Adults: A Strong Safety Net Is Not the Same as Insurance.* Series B, No. B-42. Washington, DC: The Urban Institute.

Holahan, John, Lisa Dubay, and Genevieve Kenney. 2003a. Which Children Are Still Uninsured and Why. *The Future of Children* 13(1):55-80.

Holahan, John, Catherine Hoffman, and Marie Wang. 2003b. *The New Middle-Class of Uninsured Americans —Is It Real?* Issue Paper No.4090. Washington, DC: The Kaiser Commission on Medicaid and the Uninsured.

Holahan, John, Alan Weil, and Joshua M. Wiener. 2003c. *Federalism and Health Policy.* Washington, DC: The Urban Institute.

Holahan, John, Joshua M. Wiener, Randall R. Bovbjerg, Barbara A. Ormond, et al. 2003d. *The State Fiscal Crisis and Medicaid: Will Health Programs Be Major Budget Targets?* Washington, DC: The Henry J. Kaiser Family Foundation.

Holl, Jane L., Peter G. Szilagyi, Lance E. Rodewald, Robert S. Byrd, et al. 1995. Profile of Uninsured Children in the United States. *Archives of Pediatrics and Adolescent Medicine* 149(4):398-406.

Homan, Rick K., and Carol C. Korenbrot. 1998. Explaining Variation in Birth Outcomes of Medicaid-Eligible Women with Variation in the Adequacy of Prenatal Support Services. *Medical Care* 36(2):190-201.

Howell, Embry. 2001. The Impact of the Medicaid Expansions for Pregnant Women. *Medical Care Research and Review* 58(1):3-30.

Howell, Embry, Ian Hill, and Heidi Kapustka. 2002. *SCHIP Dodges the First Budget Axe.* Health Policy On-Line, No. 3. Washington, DC: The Urban Institute.

Hurley, Jeremiah. 2000. An Overview of the Normative Economics of the Health Sector. Pp. 56-110 in: *Handbook of Health Economics*, A.J. Culyer and Joseph P. Newhouse, eds. New York: Elsevier Science.

Huttin, Christine, John F. Moeller, and Randall S. Stafford. 2000. Patterns and Costs for Hypertension Treatment in the United States. *Clinical Drug Investigation* 20(3):181-195.

Ibarra, Irene. 2002. *Covering the Uninsured in Alameda County. The Alameda Alliance.* February 28, 2002 San Francisco Committee meeting. Unpublished presentation before the IOM Committee on the Consequences of Uninsurance, San Francisco.

Ingram, Carol, Myron Levin, and Gregg Jones. 2003. Legislature OKs Small Business Health Coverage. *Los Angeles Times.* September 14, 2003.

Institute of Medicine (IOM). 1990. *Medicine: A Strategy for Quality Assurance.* Washington, DC: National Academy Press.

———. 2000. *Calling the Shots: Immunization Finance Policies and Practices.* Washington, DC: National Academy Press.

———. 2001a. *Coverage Matters: Insurance and Health Care.* Washington, DC: National Academy Press.

———. 2001b. *Crossing the Quality Chasm: A Health System for the 21st Century.* Washington, DC: National Academy Press.

———. 2002a. *Care Without Coverage: Too Little, Too Late.* Washington, DC: The National Academies Press.

———. 2002b. *Health Insurance Is a Family Matter.* Washington, DC: The National Academies Press.

———. 2003a. *A Shared Destiny: Community Effects of Uninsurance.* Washington, DC: The National Academies Press.

———. 2003b. *Hidden Costs, Value Lost: Uninsurance in America.* Washington, DC: The National Academies Press.

———. 2003c. *The Future of the Public's Health in the 21st Century.* Washington, DC: The National Academies Press.

Jacobs, Lawrence, Theodore Marmor, and Jonathan Oberlander. 1999. The Oregon Health Plan and the Political Paradox of Rationing: What Advocates and Critics Have Claimed and What Oregon Did. *Journal of Health Politics, Policy and Law* 24(1):161-180.

Jacoby, Melissa G., Teresa A. Sullivan, and Elizabeth Warren. 2000. Medical Problems and Bankruptcy Filings. *Norton's Bankruptcy Adviser.*

Jenny, Nicholas W., and Cecilia Ferradino. 2003. *State Budgetary Assumptions in 2003 States Cautiously Projecting Recovery.* State Fiscal Brief No. 68. New York: The Nelson A. Rockefeller Institute of Government.

Jensen, Gail A., and Michael A. Morrisey. 2003. Self-Insured Employer-Sponsored Health Plans and the Regulation of Managed Care. Detroit: Wayne State University, unpublished ms.

Johnson, Richard W., Marilyn M. Moon, and Amy J. Davidoff. 2002. *A Medicare Buy-In for the Near-Elderly: Design Issues and Potential Effects on Coverage.* Washington, DC: The Urban Institute.

Joint Committee on Taxation. 2001. *Estimates of Federal Tax Expenditures for Fiscal Years 2001-2005.* Washington, DC: U.S. Government Printing Office.

Kahn III, Charles N., and Ronald F. Pollack. 2001. Building a Consensus for Expanding Health Coverage. *Health Affairs* 20(1):40-48.

Kaiser Commission on Medicaid and the Uninsured (KCMU). 2002a. *Medicaid Matters for America's Families.* Accessed April 2, 2003. Available at: http://www.kcmu.org.

———. 2002b. *The New Medicaid and CHIP Waiver Initiatives.* Washington, DC: The Henry J. Kaiser Family Foundation.

———. 2003a. *Medicaid: Fiscal Challenges to Coverage.* Washington, DC: The Kaiser Commission on Medicaid and the Uninsured.

———. 2003b. *The Medicaid Program at a Glance.* Accessed April 30, 2003. Available at: http://www.kcmu.org.

———. 2003c. *State Budget Constraints: The Impact of Medicaid.* Washington, DC: The Kaiser Commission on Medicaid and the Uninsured.

———. 2003d. *State Health Facts Online. Hawaii.* Accessed October 1, 2003. Available at: http://www.statehealthfacts.kff.org/cgi-bin/healthfacts.cgi?action=profile&area=Hawaii.

———. 2003e. *State Health Facts Online. Massachusetts.* Accessed October 1, 2003. Available at: http://www.statehealthfacts.kff.org/cgi-bin/healthfacts.cgi?action=profile&area=Massachusetts.

————. 2003f. *State Health Facts Online. Minnesota.* Accessed October 1, 2003. Available at: http://www.statehealthfacts.kff.org/cgi-bin/healthfacts.cgi?action=profile&area=Minnesota.

————. 2003g. *State Health Facts Online. Oregon.* Accessed October 1, 2003. Available at: http://www.statehealthfacts.kff.org/cgi-bin/healthfacts.cgi?action=profile&area=Oregon.

————. 2003h. *State Health Facts Online. Tennessee.* Accessed October 1, 2003. Available at: http://www.statehealthfacts.kff.org/cgi-bin/healthfacts.cgi?action=profile&area=Tennessee.

Kaiser Family Foundation and the Health Research and Educational Trust (Kaiser/HRET). 2003. *Employer Health Benefits. 2003 Annual Survey.* Washington, DC: The Henry J. Kaiser Family Foundation.

Kausz, Annamaria T., Gregorio T. Obrador, Pradeep Arora, Robin Ruthazer, et al. 2000. Late Initiation of Dialysis Among Women and Ethnic Minorities in the United States. *Journal of the American Society of Nephrology* 11(12):2351-2357.

Keane, Christopher, John Marx, and Edmund Ricci. 2001. *Local Health Departments' Changing Role in Provision and Assurance of Safety Net Services.* Accessed December 2, 2002. Available at: http://www.hrsa.gov/financeMC/LHDabstract.pdf.

Kenney, Genevieve, Jennifer Haley, and Alexandra Tebay. 2003. *Children's Insurance Coverage and Service Use Improve.* Snapshots of America's Families III. Washington, DC: The Urban Institute.

Kohn, Linda, Janet M. Corrigan, and Molla S. Donaldson (eds.). 2000. *To Err Is Human. Building a Safer Health System.* Washington, DC: National Academy Press.

Kronick, Richard P. 2002. *UCSD's Evaluation of the FOCUS Program.* February 28, 2002 San Francisco Committee meeting. Unpublished presentation before the IOM Committee on the Consequences of Uninsurance.

Krueger, Alan B., and Uwe Reinhardt. 1994. The Economics of Employer Versus Individual Mandates. *Health Affairs* 13(2):34-53.

Ku, Leighton. 2003. *State Fiscal Relief Provides an Opportunity to Safeguard Medicaid Budgets.* Washington, DC: Center on Budget and Policy Priorities.

Ku, Leighton, and Shannon Blaney. 2000. *Health Coverage for Legal Immigrant Children: New Census Data Highlight Importance of Restoring Medicaid and SCHIP Coverage.* Washington, DC: Center on Budget and Policy Priorities.

Ku, Leighton, and Matthew Broaddus. 2000. *The Importance of Family-Based Insurance Expansions: New Research Findings About State Health Reforms.* Washington, DC: Center on Budget and Policy Priorities.

Ku, Leighton, and Donna C. Ross. 2002. *Staying Covered: The Importance of Retaining Health Insurance for Low-Income Families.* Pub. 586. New York: The Commonwealth Fund.

Kuttner, Hanns, and Catherine McLaughlin. 2003, May 8-9. *The Joint Dynamics of Employment and Health Insurance.* Unpublished paper presented at the Health Policy and the Underserved Conference, Washington, DC.

Lagnado, Lucette. 2003. *House Panel Begins Inquiry into Hospital Billing Practices.* Accessed July 18, 2003. Available at: http://online.wsj.com.

Lambrew, Jeanne. 2001. *How the Slowing U.S. Economy Threatens Employer-Based Health Insurance.* Pub. No. 511. New York: The Commonwealth Fund.

Lave, Judith R., Christopher R. Keane, J. L. Chyongchiou, et al. 1998. The Impact of Lack of Health Insurance on Children. *Journal of Health and Social Policy* 10(2):57-73.

Law, Sylvia A. 2000. Health Care in Hawaii: An Agenda for Research and Reform. *American Journal of Law & Medicine* 26(2-3):205-223.

Lazarus, William, Brady Foust, and Ben Hitt. 2000. *The Florida Health Insurance Study. Volume 6: The Small Area Analysis.* Tallahassee: The State of Florida, Agency for Health Care Administration.

Leape, Lucian L., L. H. Hilborne, R. Bell, C. Kamberg, and Robert H. Brook. 1999. Underuse of Cardiac Procedures: Do Women, Ethnic Minorities, and the Uninsured Fail to Receive Needed Revascularization? *Annals of Internal Medicine* 130(3):183-192.

Lee-Feldstein, Anna, Paul J. Feldstein, Thomas Buchmuller, and Gale Katterhagen. 2000. The Relationship of HMOs, Health Insurance, and Delivery Systems to Breast Cancer Outcomes. *Medical Care* 38(7):705-718.

Leichter, Howard M. 1999. Oregon's Bold Experiment: Whatever Happened to Rationing? *Journal of Health Politics, Policy and Law* 24(1):147-160.

Levit, Katherine R., Gary L. Olin, and Suzanne W. Letsch. 1992. Americans' Health Insurance Coverage, 1980-91. *Health Care Financing Review* 14(1):31-57.

Levy, Helen, and Thomas DeLiere. 2002. *What Do People Buy When They Don't Buy Health Insurance?* Accessed June 27, 2002. Available at: http://www.chas.chicago.edu/events/wspapers/05302002.pdf.

Lewin Group. 2002. *Emergency Department Overload: A Growing Crisis.* Washington, DC: American Hospital Association, American College of Emergency Physicians.

Lewin, Marion E., and Stuart Altman (eds.). 2000. *America's Health Care Safety Net: Intact But Endangered.* Washington, DC: National Academy Press.

Lewis, Irving. 1983. Evolution of Federal Policy on Access to Health Care, 1965-1980. *Bulletin of the New York Academy of Medicine* 59(1):9-20.

Li, Guohua, and Griffin Davis. 2001. Insurance Status and Survival Outcome in Pediatric Trauma. *Academic Emergency Medicine* 8(5):517.

Long, Sharon K. 2003. *Hardship Among the Uninsured: Choosing Among Food, Housing, and Health Insurance.* Series B, No. B-54. Washington, DC: The Urban Institute.

Looker, Anne C., Peter R. Dallman, Margaret D. Carroll, Elaine W. Gunter, et al. 1997. Prevalence of Iron Deficiency in the United States. *Journal of the American Medical Association* 277(12):973-976.

Loprest, Pamela, and Cori Uccello. 1997. *Uninsured Older Adults: Implications for Changing Medicare Eligibility.* New York: The Commonwealth Fund.

LoSasso, Anthony T., and Thomas C. Buchmueller. 2002. *The Effect of the State Children's Health Insurance Program on Health Insurance Coverage.* NBER Working Paper No. 9405. Cambridge, MA: National Bureau of Economic Research.

Lurie, Nicole, N. B. Ward, Martin F. Shapiro, and Robert H. Brook. 1984. Termination from Medi-Cal: Does It Affect Health? *New England Journal of Medicine* 311(7):480-484.

———. 1986. Termination of Medi-Cal Benefits: A Followup Study One Year Later. *New England Journal of Medicine* 314(19):1266-1268.

Madrian, Brigitte C. 1994. Employment-Based Health Insurance and Job Mobility: Is There Evidence of Job-Lock? *The Quarterly Journal of Economics* 109:27-54.

Maioni, Antonia. 1998. *Parting at the Crossroads: The Emergence of Health Insurance in the United States and Canada.* Princeton, NJ: Princeton University Press.

Mann, Cindy. 2002. *The New Medicaid and CHIP Waiver Initiatives.* Pub. No. 4028. Washington, DC: The Henry J. Kaiser Family Foundation.

Mann, Cindy, Diane Rowland, and Rachel Garfield. 2003. Historical Overview of Children's Health Care Coverage. *The Future of Children* 13(1):31-54.

Marmor, Theodore. 1973. *The Politics of Medicare.* Chicago: Aldine.

Marmor, Theodore R., and Morris L. Barer. 1997. The Politics of Universal Health Insurance: Lessons for and from the 1990s. Pp. 306-322 in: *Health Politics and Policy,* 3rd ed., Theodore J. Litman and Leonard S. Robins, eds. Washington, DC: Delmar Publishers.

Marquis, M. Susan, and Stephen H. Long. 1997. Federalism and Health System Reform. Prospects for State Action. *Journal of the American Medical Association* 278(6):514-517.

———. 2002. The Role of Public Insurance and the Public Delivery System in Improving Health Outcomes for Low-Income Pregnant Women. *Medical Care* 40(11):1048-59.

McAlearney, John S. 2002. The Financial Performance of Community Health Centers, 1996-1999. *Health Affairs* 21(2):219-225.

McAlpine, Donna D., and David Mechanic. 2000. Utilization of Specialty Mental Health Care Among Persons with Severe Mental Illness: The Roles of Demographics, Need, Insurance, and Risk. *Health Services Research* 35(1):277-282.

McArdle, Frank B. 1994. How Would Business React to an Employer Mandate? *Health Affairs* 13(2):69-83.

McBride, Timothy D. 1997. Uninsured Spells of the Poor: Prevalence and Duration. *Health Care Financing* 19(1):145-160.

McCormick, Marie C., Robin M. Weinick, Anne Elixhauser, Marie N. Stagnitti, et al. 2001. Annual Report on Access to and Utilization of Health Care for Children and Youth in the United States–2000. *Ambulatory Pediatrics* 1(1):3-15.

McNichol, Liz. 2003. *The State Fiscal Crisis: Extent, Causes, and Responses.* Washington, DC: Center on Budget and Policy Priorities.

Merlis, Mark. 2001. *Family Out-of-Pocket Spending on Health Services: A Continuing Source of Financial Insecurity.* Pub. No. 509. New York: The Commonwealth Fund.

Meyer, Jack A., and Larry S. Stepnick. 2002. *Portability of Coverage: HIPAA and COBRA.* Issue Brief No. 569. New York: The Commonwealth Fund.

Meyer, Jack A., and Elliot K. Wicks (eds). 2001. *Covering America: Real Remedies for the Uninsured.* Washington, DC: Economic and Social Research Institute.

Meyer, Jack A., and Elliot K. Wicks (eds.). 2002. *Covering America: Real Remedies for the Uninsured.* Vol. 2. Washington, DC: Economic and Social Research Institute.

MGT of America. 2002. *Medical Emergency: Costs of Uncompensated Care in Southwest Border Counties.* Washington, DC: United States/Mexico Border Counties Coalition.

Miller, Sara B. 2003. Probing Disparity in Healthcare Bills. *Christian Science Monitor.* Accessed May 20, 2003. Available at: http://www.csmonitor.com/2003/0519/p16s01-wmcn.htm.

Mills, Robert J. 2001. *Health Insurance Coverage: 2000. Current Population Reports.* P60-215. Washington, DC: U.S. Census Bureau.

———. 2002. *Health Insurance Coverage: 2001. Current Population Reports.* P60-220. Washington, DC: U.S. Census Bureau.

Mills, Robert J., and Shailesh Bhandari. 2003. *Health Insurance Coverage in the United States: 2002.* Current Population Reports. P60-223. Washington, DC: U.S. Census Bureau.

Morone, James A. 2002. Medicare for All. Pp. 63-74 in: *Covering America: Real Remedies for the Uninsured.* Jack A. Meyer and Elliot K. Wicks, eds. Washington, DC: Economic and Social Research Institute.

Murphy, Kevin M., and Robert Topel. 1999. *The Economic Value of Medical Research.* Chicago: University of Chicago.

Musgrove, Philip. 2003. Judging Health Sytems: Reflections on WHO's Methods. *The Lancet* 361:817-820.

Nathanson, Melanie, and Leighton Ku. 2003. *Proposed State Medicaid Cuts Would Jeopardize Health Insurance Coverage for 1.7 Million People: An Update.* Washington, DC: Center on Budget and Policy Priorities.

National Center for Health Statistics. 2002. Table 23. *Infant Mortality Rates, Fetal Mortality Rates, and Perinatal Mortality Rates, According to Race: United States, Selected Years 1950-99.* Accessed April 16, 2003. Available at: http://www.cdc.gov/nchs/products/pubs/pubd/hus/listables.pdf# Mortality.

National Governors Association. 2003. *Governors to Meet with President, Cabinet Officials and Congressional Leaders During NGA Winter Meeting.* Accessed April 17, 2003. Available at: http://www.nga.org/nga/newsroom/pressreleasedetailprint/1,1422,5079,00.html.

Needleman, Jack, and Darrell J. Gaskin. 2003. The Impact of Uninsured Discharges on the Availability of Hospital Services and Hospital Margins in Rural Areas. Pp. 221-35 in: *A Shared Destiny: Community Effects of Uninsurance,* Institute of Medicine. Washington, DC: The National Academies Press.

Neubauer, Deane. 1993. State Model: Hawaii. A Pioneer In Health System Reform. *Health Affairs* 12(2):31-39.

Newacheck, Paul W., Bonnie Strickland, Jack P. Shonkoff, James M. Perrin, et al. 1998a. An Epidemiologic Profile of Children with Special Health Care Needs. *Pediatrics* 102(1):117-123.

Newacheck, Paul W., Jeffrey J. Stoddard, Dana C. Hughes, and Michelle Pearl. 1998b. Health Insurance and Access to Primary Care for Children. *New England Journal of Medicine* 338(8):513-518.

Newacheck, Paul W., Claire D. Brindis, Courtney U. Cart, Kristin Marchi, et al. 1999. Adolescent Health Insurance Coverage: Recent Changes and Access to Care. *Pediatrics* 104(2, Pt. 1 of 2):195-202.

Newhouse, Joseph P., and The Insurance Experiment Group. 1993. *Free for All? Lessons from the RAND Health Insurance Experiment.* Cambridge, MA: Harvard University Press.

Nichols, Len M., and Linda J. Blumberg. 1998. A Different Kind of New Federalism? The Health Insurance Portability and Accountability Act of 1996. *Health Affairs* 17(3):25-42.

Norato, Joseph F. 1997. National Health Care Reform and a Single-Payer System: Messiah or Pariah? *Journal of Health and Human Services Administration* 19(3):341-356.

Numbers, Ronald, 1978. *Almost Persuaded. American Physicians and Compulsory Health Insurance, 1912-1920.* Baltimore, MD: Johns Hopkins University Press.

Numbers, Ronald L. 1985. The Third Party: Health Insurance in America. Pp. 233-247 in: *Sickness and Health in America: Readings in the History of Medicine and Public Health,* 2nd ed., Judith Leavitt and Ronald Numbers, eds. Madison: University of Wisconsin Press.

Oberlander, Jonathan. 2003. The Politics of Health Reform: Why Do Bad Things Happen to Good Plans? *Health Affairs* Web Exclusive:W3-391-W3-404.

O'Connor, Patrick J., Jay Desai, William A. Rush, Linda Cherney, et al. 1998. Is Having a Regular Provider of Diabetes Care Related to Intensity of Care and Glycemic Control? *Journal of Family Practice* 47(4):290-297.

Oliver, Thomas R., and Pamela Paul-Shaheen. 1997. Translating Ideas into Actions: Entrepreneurial Leadership in State Health Care Reforms. *Journal of Health Politics, Policy and Law* 22(3):721-788.

Organization for Economic Cooperation and Development (OECD). 2002. *OECD Health Data 2002: A Comparative Analysis of Twenty-Nine Countries,* 4th ed. CD-ROM. Paris: OECD.

Orenstein, Charles, and Sue Fox. 2003. California and Maine Laws May Be Models for Action on the Uninsured. Without Federal Action, States Take the Lead. *Los Angeles Times.* September 15, 2003.

Ormond, Barbara A., Susan Wallin, and Susan M. Goldenson. 2000. *Supporting the Rural Health Care Safety Net.* Occasional Paper No. 36. Washington, DC: The Urban Institute.

Overpeck, Mary D., Diane H. Jones, Ann C. Truble, et al. 1997. Socioeconomic and Racial/Ethnic Factors Affecting Non-Fatal Medically Attended Injury Rates in U.S. Children. *Injury Prevention* 3:272-276.

Pappas, Gregory, Wilbur C. Hadden, Lola Jean Kozak, and Gail F. Fisher. 1997. Potentially Avoidable Hospitalizations: Inequities in Rates Between US Socioeconomic Groups. *American Journal of Public Health* 87(5):811-816.

Paul-Shaheen, Pamela A. 1998. The States and Health Care Reform: The Road Traveled and Lessons Learned from Seven That Took the Lead. *Journal of Health Politics, Policy and Law* 23(2):319-361.

Pauly, Mark V., and Bradley Herring. 2001. Expanding Coverage Via Tax Credits: Trade-Offs and Outcomes. *Health Affairs* 20(1):9-26.

Pauly, Mark V., and Len M. Nichols. 2002. The Nongroup Health Insurance Market: Short on Facts, Long on Opinions and Policy Disputes. *Health Affairs* Web Exclusive:W325-W343.

Penson, David F., Marcia L. Stoddard, David J. Pasta, Deborah P. Lubeck, et al. 2001. The Association Between Socioeconomic Status, Health Insurance Coverage, and Quality of Life in Men with Prostate Cancer. *Journal of Clinical Epidemiology* 54(4):350-358.

Perkins, Carin, William E. Wright, Mark Allen, Steven J. Samuels, et al. 2001. Breast Cancer Stage at Diagnosis in Relation to Duration of Medicaid Enrollment. *Medical Care* 39(11):1224-1233.

Perry, Michael. 2002. *New York's Disaster Relief Medicaid: Insights and Implications for Covering Low-Income People*. Washington, DC: The Kaiser Commission on Medicaid and the Uninsured, in collaboration with the United Hospital Fund.

Phibbs, C. S., D. H. Mark, H. S. Luft, D. J. Peltzman-Rennie, et al. 1993. Choice of Hospital for Delivery: A Comparison of High-Risk and Low-Risk Women. *Health Services Research* 28(2): 201-222.

Poen, Monte M. 1979. *Harry S. Truman Versus the Medical Lobby: The Genesis of Medicare*. Columbia: University of Missouri Press.

Pollitz, Karen, Richard Sorian, and Kathy Thomas. 2001. *How Accessible is Individual Health Insurance for Consumers in Less-Than-Perfect Health?* Accessed June 20, 2001. Available at: http://www.kff.org.

Ponce, Ninez, Tomiko Conner, B. P. Barrera, and Dong Suh. 2001. *Advancing Universal Health Insurance Coverage in Alameda County: Results of the County of Alameda Uninsured Survey*. Los Angeles: UCLA Center for Health Policy Research and Community Voices Project-Oakland.

Powell-Griner, Eve, Julie Bolen, and Shayne Bland. 1999. Health Care Coverage and Use of Preventive Services Among the Near Elderly in the United States. *American Journal of Public Health* 89(6):882-886.

Quinn, Kevin, Cathy Schoen, and Louisa Buatti. 2000. *On Their Own: Young Adults Living Without Health Insurance*. Pub. No. 391. New York: The Commonwealth Fund, Task Force on the Future of Health Insurance for Working Americans.

Rabinowitz, Jonathan, Evelyn Bromet, Janet Lavelle, G. Carlson, et al. 1998. Relationship Between Type of Insurance and Care During Early Course of Psychosis. *American Journal of Psychiatry* 155(10):1392-1397.

Rabinowitz, Jonathan, Evelyn J. Bromet, Janet Lavelle, Kimberly J. Hornak, et al. 2001. Changes in Insurance Coverage and Extent of Care During the Two Years After First Hospitalization for a Psychotic Disorder. *Psychiatric Services* 52(1):87-91.

Reed, Marie C., Peter J. Cunningham, and Jeffrey J. Stoddard. 2001. *Physicians Pulling Back from Charity Care*. Issue Brief. Washington, DC: Center for Studying Health System Change 42:1-4.

Reynolds, P. Preston. 1997. The Federal Government's Use of Title VI and Medicare to Racially Integrate Hospitals in the United States, 1963 Through 1967. *American Journal of Public Health* 87(11):1850-1858.

Rhoades, Jeffrey A., and Joel W.Cohen. 2003. *The Uninsured in America –1996-2002. Estimates for the Civilian Noninstitutionalized Population Under Age 65*. Statistical Brief No. 24. Rockville, MD: Agency for Healthcare Research and Quality.

Rodewald, Lance E., Peter G. Szilagyi, Jane Holl, Laura R. Shone, et al. 1997. Health Insurance for Low-Income Working Families. *Archives of Pediatric and Adolescent Medicine* 151(8):798-803.

Roetzheim, Richard G., Naazneen Pal, Colleen Tennant, Lydia Voti, et al. 1999. Effects of Health Insurance and Race on Early Detection of Cancer. *Journal of the National Cancer Institute* 91(16):1409-1415.

Roetzheim, Richard G., Eduardo C. Gonzalez, Jeanne M. Ferrante, Naazneen Pal, et al. 2000a. Effects of Health Insurance and Race on Breast Carcinoma Treatments and Outcomes. *Cancer* 89(11):2202-2213.

Roetzheim, Richard G., Naazneen Pal, Eduardo C. Gonzalez, Jeanne M. Ferrante, Daniel J. Van Durme, and Jeffrey P. Krischer. 2000b. Effects of Health Insurance and Race on Colorectal Cancer Treatments and Outcomes. *American Journal of Public Health* 90(11):1746-1754.

Rosenbaum, Sara. 2000. *Medicaid Eligibility and Citizenship Status: Policy Implications for Immigrant Populations*. Pub. No. 2201. Washington, DC: The Kaiser Commission on Medicaid and the Uninsured.

Rosenbaum, Sara, and Barbara Smith. 2001. *Policy Brief #1: State SCHIP Design and the Right to Coverage*. SCHIP Policy Studies Project. Washington, DC: The George Washington University, Center for Health Services Research and Policy.

Rosenbaum, Sara, Jeanne Lambrew, Peter Shin, Marsha Regenstein, et al. 2002. *Health Coverage in Massachusetts: Far to Go, Farther to Fall. Report for the Blue Cross Blue Shield of Massachusetts Foundation.* Washington, DC: The George Washington University, Center for Health Services Research and Policy.

Ross, Donna Cohen, and Laura Cox. 2003. *Preserving Recent Progress on Health Coverage for Children and Families: New Tensions Emerge: A 50 State Update on Eligibility, Enrollment, Renewal and Cost-Sharing Practices in Medicaid and SCHIP.* Pub. No. 4125. Washington, DC: The Kaiser Commission on Medicaid and the Uninsured.

Rowland, Diane. 2003. *State Fiscal Pressures and Medicaid.* Washington, DC: The Kaiser Commission on Medicaid and the Uninsured.

Rundle, Rhoda. 2003. Sacramento Passes Bill Requiring Companies to Offer Health Benefit. *Wall Street Journal.* September 15, 2003.

Russakoff, Dale. 2001. Out of Tragedy, N.Y. Finds Way to Treat Medicaid Need: Streamlined Post-Crisis Process Draws Record Enrollment Through a Multilingual Grapevine. *New York Times,* November 26, 2001. p. A02.

Sacks, Heather, Todd Kutyla, and Sharon Silow-Carroll. 2002. *Toward Comprehensive Health Coverage for All: Summaries of 20 State Planning Grants From the U.S. Health Resources and Services Administration.* Pub. No. 4046. New York: The Commonwealth Fund.

Salganicoff, Alina, and Roberta Wyn. 1999. Access to Care for Low-Income Women: The Impact of Medicaid. *Journal of Health Care for the Poor and Underserved* 10(4):453-467.

Schlesinger, Mark, and Karl Kronebusch. 1990. The Failure of Prenatal Care Policy for the Poor. *Health Affairs* 9(4):91-111.

Schneider, Andy. 2002. *The Medicaid Resource Book.* Washington, DC: The Kaiser Commission on Medicaid and the Uninsured.

Shapiro, Martin F., Sally C. Morton, Daniel F. McCaffrey, et al. 1999. Variations in the Care of HIV-Infected Adults in the United States. *Journal of the American Medical Association* 281(24):2305-2315.

Shea, Steven, Dawn Misra, Martin Ehrlich, et al. 1992a. Correlates of Nonadherence to Hypertension Treatment in an Inner-City Minority Population. *American Journal of Public Health* 82(12):1607-1612.

———. 1992b. Predisposing Factors for Severe, Uncontrolled Hypertension in an Inner-City Minority Population. *New England Journal of Medicine* 327(11):776-781.

Sheils, John F., Gary J. Young, and Robert J. Rubin. 1992. O Canada: Do We Expect Too Much from Its Health System? *Health Affairs* 11(1):7-20.

Shi, Leiyu. 2000. Vulnerable Populations and Health Insurance. *Medical Care Research and Review* 57(1):110-134.

———. 2001. The Convergence of Vulnerable Characteristics and Health Insurance in the US. *Social Science and Medicine* 53(4):519-529.

Short, Pamela F. 2001. *Counting and Characterizing the Uninsured.* Accessed May 6, 2003. Available at: http://www.umich.edu/~eriu/pdf/wp2.pdf.

Short, Pamela F., and Vicki A. Freedman. 1998. Single Women and the Dynamics of Medicaid. *Health Services Research* 33(5):1309-1336.

Short, Pamela F., Dennis G. Shea, and M. P. Powell. 2001. *Health Insurance on the Way to Medicare: Is Special Government Assistance Warranted?* New York: The Commonwealth Fund.

Silow-Carroll, Sharon, Stephanie E. Anthony, and Jack A. Meyer. 2000. *State and Local Initiatives to Enhance Health Coverage for the Working Uninsured.* Pub. No. 424. New York: The Commonwealth Fund.

Silow-Carroll, Sharon, Emily K. Waldman, and Jack A. Meyer. 2001. *Expanding Employment-Based Health Coverage: Lessons from Six State and Local Programs.* Pub. No. 445. New York: The Commonwealth Fund.

Skeels, Michael R. 1994. The Oregon Health Plan and Public Health. *Journal of Health & Social Policy* 6(1):21-31.

Skocpol, Theda. 1996. *Boomerang. Clinton's Health Security Effort and the Turn Against Government in U.S. Politics.* New York: W.W. Norton and Company.

Smedley, Brian D., and S. Leonard Syme (eds.). 2000. *Promoting Health: Intervention Strategies from Social and Behavioral Research.* Washington, DC: National Academy Press.

Smedley, Brian D., Adrienne Y. Stith, and Alan R. Nelson (eds.). 2002. *Unequal Treatment: Confronting Racial and Ethnic Disparities in Health Care.* Washington, DC: National Academies Press.

Smith, Vernon, and Eileen Ellis. 2002. *Medicaid Budgets Under Stress: Survey Findings for State Fiscal Years 2000, 2001, 2002.* Pub. No. 4019. Washington, DC: The Kaiser Commission on Medicaid and the Uninsured.

Smith, Vernon, Eileen Ellis, Kathy Gifford, Rekha Ramesh, et al. 2002. *Medicaid Spending Growth: Results from a 2002 Survey.* Pub. No. 4064. Washington, DC: The Henry J. Kaiser Family Foundation.

Smith, Vernon, Rekha Ramesh, Kathy Gifford, Eileen Ellis, et al. 2003. *States Respond to Fiscal Pressure: State Medicaid Spending Growth and Cost Containment in Fiscal Years 2003 and 2004. Results from a 50-State Survey.* Washington, DC: The Kaiser Commission on Medicaid and the Uninsured.

Somers, Herman Miles, and Anne Ramsay Somers. 1961. *Doctors, Patients, and Health Insurance. The Organization and Financing of Medical Care.* Garden City, NY: Anchor Books/Doubleday & Company.

Sorlie, Paul D., Norman J. Johnson., Eric Backlund, and Douglas D. Bradham. 1994. Mortality in the Uninsured Compared with That in Persons with Public and Private Health Insurance. *Archives of Internal Medicine* 154(21):2409-2416.

Starfield, Barbara. 2000. Is US Health Really the Best in the World? *Journal of the American Medical Association* 284(4):483-485.

Starr, Paul. 1982. *The Social Transformation of American Medicine.* New York: Basic Books.

———. 1992. *The Logic of Health Care Reform.* Knoxville, TN: Whittle Direct Books.

State of Hawaii. 2002. *Hawaii Health Survey (HHS).* Accessed September 10, 2003. Available at: http://www.state.hi.us/doh/stats/surveys/hhs.html.

Steinmo, Sven, and Jon Watts. 1995. It's the Institutions, Stupid! Why Comprehensive National Health Insurance Always Fails in America. *Journal of Health Policy, Politics and Law* 20(2):329-372.

Steuerle, C. Eugene. 1994. Implementing Employer and Individual Mandates. *Health Affairs* 13(2):54-68.

Stevens, Rosemary. 1989. *In Sickness and in Wealth: America's Hospitals in the Twentieth Century.* New York: Basic Books.

Sturm, Roland, and Kenneth B. Wells. 1995. How Can Care for Depression Become More Cost-Effective? *Journal of the American Medical Association* 273(1):51-58.

Sutton, Janet, Bonnie B. Blanchfield, Andrew Singer, and Meredith J. Milet. 2001. *Is the Rural Safety Net at Risk? Analyses of Charity and Uncompensated Care Provided By Rural Hospitals in Washington, West Virginia, Texas, Iowa, and Vermont.* Bethesda, MD: The Project HOPE Walsh Center for Rural Health Analysis.

Szalavitz, Maia. 2002. *Disaster Relief Medicaid.* Accessed July 7, 2003. Available at: http://www.gothamgazette.com/health/apr.02.shtml.

Taylor, Amy K., Joel W. Cohen, and Steven R. Machlin. 2001. *Unpublished Tables. Being Uninsured in 1996 Compared to 1987: How Has the Experience of the Uninsured Changed Over Time?* Center for Cost and Financing Studies. Rockville, MD: Agency for Healthcare Research and Quality.

Taylor, Todd B. 2001. Emergency Services Crisis of 2000—The Arizona Experience. *Academic Emergency Medicine* 8(11):1107-1108.

Technological Change in Health Care (TECH) Research Network. 2001. *Technological Change Around the World: Evidence from Heart Attack Care.* 20(3):25-42.

Thorpe, Kenneth E., and Curtis S. Florence. 1999. Why Are Workers Uninsured? Employer-Sponsored Health Insurance in 1997. *Health Affairs* 18(2):213-218.

Ullman, Frank C., and Ian Hill. 2001. Eligibility Under State Children's Health Insurance Programs. *American Journal of Public Health* 91(9):1449-1451.

U.S. Bureau of Labor Statistics. 2003a. *Consumer Price Indexes.* Accessed April 17, 2003. Available at: http://www.bls.gov/cpi/home.htm.

———. 2003b. *Labor Force Statistics from the Current Population Survey.* Accessed April 17, 2003. Available at: http://data.bls.gov/servlet/SurveyOutputServlet.

U.S. Census Bureau. 2001. *Money Income in the United States: 2000.* Washington, DC: U.S. Government Printing Office.

———. 2003a. *Current Population Survey. Annual Demographic Survey. March Supplement. Table HI01. Health Insurance Coverage Status and Type of Coverage by Selected Characteristics: 2002. All Races.* Accessed October 3, 2003. Available at: http://ferret.bls.census.gov/macro/032003/health/h01_001.htm.

———. 2003b. *Current Population Survey. Annual Demographic Survey. March Supplement. Table HI03. Health Insurance Coverage Status and Type of Coverage by Selected Characteristics for Poor People in the Poverty Universe: 2002.* Accessed October 3, 2003. Available at: http://ferret.bls.census.gov/macro/032003/health/h03_000.htm.

———. 2003c. *Current Population Survey. Annual Demographic Survey. March Supplement. Table HI04. Health Insurance Coverage Status and Type of Coverage by Selected Characteristics for Near Poor People in the Poverty Universe: 2002.* Accessed October 3, 2003. Available at: http://ferret.bls.census.gov/macro/032003/health/h04_000.htm.

———. 2003d. *Current Population Survey. Annual Demographic Survey. March Supplement. Table HI05. Health Insurance Coverage Status and Type of Coverage by State and Age for All People: 2002.* Accessed October 3, 2003. Available at: http://ferret.bls.census.gov/macro/032003/health/h05_000.htm.

U.S. Congress. 1974. *Congressional Budget and Impoundment Control Act of 1974, PL 93-344, sec.3(3).* Washington, DC: U.S. Government Printing Office.

U.S. Department of Health and Human Services (DHHS). 2000. *Access to Health Care. Leading Health Indicator.* Accessed August 19, 2003. Available at: http://www.healthypeople.gov/document/html/uh/uh_bw/Uh_4.htm.

———. 2003. *The 2003 HHS Poverty Guidelines.* Accessed May 6, 2003. Available at: http://aspe.hhs.gov/poverty/03poverty.htm.

U.S. General Accounting Office (GAO). 1994. *Health Care In Hawaii. Implications for National Reform.* GAO/HEHS-94-68. Washington, DC.

———. 1996. *Private Health Insurance: Millions Relying on Individual Market Face Cost and Coverage Trade-Offs.* Washington, DC.

———. 2000. *Private Health Insurance: Cooperatives Offer Small Employers Plan Choice and Market Prices.* GAO/HEHS-00-49. Washington, DC.

———. 2001. *Private Health Insurance: Small Employers Continue to Face Challenges in Providing Coverage.* GAO-02-8. Washington, DC.

———. 2002. *Health Insurance: States' Protections and Programs Benefit Some Unemployed Individuals.* GAO-03-191. Washington, DC.

———. 2003. *Hospital Preparedness: Most Urban Hospitals Have Emergency Plans but Lack Certain Capacities for Bioterrorism Response.* GAO-03-924. Washington, DC.

Waldholz, Michael. 2003. Health Insurance Experiment in California Is Welcome News. *Wall Street Journal,* October 8, 2003.

Wang, Philip S., Patricia Berglund, and Ronald C. Kessler. 2000. Recent Care of Common Mental Disorders in the United States. *Journal of General Internal Medicine* 15:284-292.

Weil, Alan, and Ian Hill. 2003. The State Children's Health Insurance Program: A New Approach to Federalism. Pp. 293-324 in: *Federalism and Health Policy,* John Holahan, Alan Weil, and Joshua Wiener (eds.). Washington, DC: The Urban Institute.

Weil, Alan R. 2001a. Increments Toward What? *Health Affairs* 20(1):68-82.

———. 2001b. The Medical Security System: A Proposal to Ensure Health Insurance Coverage for All Americans. Pp. 175-192 in: *Covering America: Real Remedies for the Uninsured.* Jack A. Meyer and Elliot K. Wicks, eds. Washington, DC: Economic and Social Research Institute.

Weinick, Robin, John Billings, and Helen Burstin. 2002. What Is the Role of Primary Care in Emergency Department Overcrowding? *Overcrowded Emergency Rooms: Do We Need More Capacity or Fewer Patients?* Washington, DC: The Henry J. Kaiser Family Foundation.

Weinick, Robin M., Samuel H. Zuvekas, and Joel W. Cohen. 2000. Racial and Ethnic Differences in Access to and Use of Health Care Services, 1977 to 1996. *Medical Care Research and Review* 57(Suppl. 1):36-54.

Weis, Darlene. 1992. Uninsured Maternity Clients: A Concern for Quality. *Applied Nursing Research* 5(2):74-82.

Wicks, Elliot. 2002. *Health Insurance Purchasing Cooperatives.* Issue Brief No. 567. New York: The Commonwealth Fund.

Wicks, Elliot K. 2003a. *Issues in Coverage Expansion Design: Coping with Risk Segmentation: Challenges and Policy Options.* Washington, DC: Economic and Social Research Institute.

———. 2003b. *Issues in Coverage Design: Decision Points and Trade-Offs in Developing Comprehensive Health Coverage Reforms.* Washington, DC: Economic and Social Research Institute.

Wilensky, Gail R. 1994. Health Reform: What Will It Take to Pass? *Health Affairs* 13(1):179-191.

Wooldridge, Judith, Ian Hill, Mary Harrington, Genevieve Kenney, et al. 2003. *Interim Evaluation Report: Congressionally Mandated Evaluation of the State Children's Health Insurance Program.* Accessed March 31, 2003. Available at: http://www.dhhs.gov.

World Health Organization (WHO). 2000. *The World Health Report 2000—Health Systems: Improving Performance.* Geneva, Switzerland.

Zambrana, Ruth E., Nancy Breen, Sarah A. Fox, and Mary L. Gutierrez-Mohamed. 1999. Use of Cancer Screening Services by Hispanic Women: Analyses by Subgroup. *Preventive Medicine* 29(6 Pt. 1):466-477.

Zuckerman, Stephen, Jennifer Haley, and Matthew Fragale. 2001. *Could Subsidizing COBRA Health Insurance Coverage Help Most Low-Income Unemployed?* Washington, DC: The Urban Institute.

Zuvekas, Samuel H., and Robin M. Weinick. 1999. Changes in Access to Care, 1977-1996: The Role of Health Insurance. *Health Services Research* 34(1):271-279.